D0876411

Aging with a Plan

Aging with a Plan

How a Little Thought Today Can Vastly Improve Your Tomorrow

Sharona Hoffman

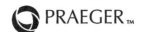

PRAEGER™

An Imprint of ABC-CLIO, LLC

Santa Barbara, California • Denver, Colorado

Library of Congress Cataloging-in-Publication Data

Hoffman, Sharona.
  Aging with a plan : how a little thought today can vastly improve your tomorrow / Sharona Hoffman.
    pages cm
  Includes bibliographical references and index.
    ISBN 978-1-4408-3890-3 (alk. paper) – ISBN 978-1-4408-3891-0 (ebook)   1. Retirement–Planning.   2. Older people–Care. I. Title.
    HQ1062.H634 2015
    332.024'014–dc23   2015001812

ISBN: 978-1-4408-3890-3
EISBN: 978-1-4408-3891-0

19 18 17 16 15   1 2 3 4 5

This book is also available on the World Wide Web as an eBook.
Visit www.abc-clio.com for details.

Praeger
An Imprint of ABC-CLIO, LLC

ABC-CLIO, LLC
130 Cremona Drive, P.O. Box 1911
Santa Barbara, California 93116-1911

This book is printed on acid-free paper ∞
Manufactured in the United States of America

In memory of my parents,
Morton and Aviva Hoffman

,

Contents

Acknowledgments

First and foremost I thank the many relatives and friends who shared their lives and their stories with me. They have taught me so much about the difficulties and triumphs that people experience at every stage, but especially when they care for elderly relatives or face their own end-of-life challenges. To my parents and mother-in-law, I am indebted not only for teaching me countless life lessons but also for their unflagging love, support, and encouragement. I will miss the three of them terribly.

Case Western Reserve University (CWRU) has been my intellectual home for over 15 years and has given me the opportunity to have an incredibly fulfilling career. I am grateful for being included among its faculty and also for financial support for this book project. A CWRU ACES Advance Opportunity Grant enabled me to do early research, and a law school summer grant and sabbatical allowed me to complete the project.

The Robert Wood Johnson Foundation selected me for a 2013 Scholar in Residence Fellowship to work with the Oregon Health Authority on the regulation of in-home care. That experience provided valuable insights into this important source of services for the elderly. During my sabbatical semester in 2014, Emory University School of Law welcomed me as a visiting scholar and supplied a beautiful office space in which it was a pleasure to work on the manuscript.

I am grateful to the ethics committee at Cleveland's University Hospitals Case Medical Center for exposing me to the complexities of numerous elder care issues and enabling me to be an active participant in discussions of treatment controversies as well as decision making for incapacitated patients without proxies. I have also learned much from staff members at a number of continuing care retirement communities that I visited and hospices that cared compassionately for my loved ones.

Several readers of early drafts provided comments that helped me improve the manuscript significantly. They are Jaime Bouvier, Naomi Cahn, Tony Moulton, and Cassandra Robertson. Jennifer Armstrong provided detailed edits and suggestions that were invaluable. Leon Gabinet spent hours with me discussing wills, trusts, and estates, and these discussions provided a strong foundation for my treatment of these matters in the book. Numerous other colleagues offered inspiration and advice and ensured that I would not lose faith in this project.

A special thank you to two Cowen Research Fellows at CWRU School of Law whose work was vital to this book: Stephanie Corley and Tracy (Yeheng) Li. Halden Schwale also provided very capable research assistance.

My thanks go also to my fabulous team of editors: Mary Bearden, Nicholle Lutz, and Nicole Azze. I am particularly grateful to my acquisition editor, Catherine LaFuente, for her enthusiasm and patience in answering my many questions.

Finally, my deepest thanks go to my husband, Andy. For the past decade, he has been a loving husband and an intellectual partner. He has made my work better and my life far richer.

Introduction

As often happened in those days, my lunchtime conversation with a colleague drifted to the subject of elder care. My husband and I had been immersed in caring for elderly relatives who were in their mid-eighties and beyond. During an 18-month period in 2013 and 2014, we lost my mother who died at the age of 84, Andy's mother who died at 93, and my father who died at 87. My friend revealed that she was coordinating care for her mother, who was in her nineties, had advanced dementia, and lived in another state. I said that sometimes I felt that our parents were lucky because at least they had us to help them, and that I have begun to worry about my own old age because Andy and I have no children. Then my friend surprised me by saying that she enjoys a very close relationship with her only son, but what she fears most about aging is that he will come to dread visiting her and will consider contact with her to be an unwelcome obligation. Having a devoted child, therefore, was hardly a comfort when she contemplated her later years.

This book, *Aging with a Plan*, began with my own efforts to identify strategies that I could adopt to minimize the potential pitfalls of aging. It also grew out of a desire to help my contemporaries who may find themselves suddenly immersed in caring for elderly relatives, a sometimes overwhelming task for which little in life prepares us. It is meant to be a concise but comprehensive resource for middle-aged people who have much to gain from thinking ahead.

In the process of researching and writing, I have learned a great deal. Too many elderly individuals refuse needed professional care giving because of its costs and the loss of autonomy it involves; some undergo aggressive medical interventions that exacerbate rather than improve their conditions; and others end up in institutional settings that are inadequately staffed and whose services at times border on neglect. Yet I have also found much reassurance.

I am convinced that many other people in their forties, fifties, and early sixties can benefit from the knowledge I gained and from investing some effort in planning for their old age as well as for that of their loved ones. As I have learned the hard way, in the midst of crisis, it is very difficult to make the best possible decisions if you have never contemplated the matter at hand.

WHY I WROTE THE BOOK

"Shoot me before I get to be like my [mother, aunt, grandfather]" is an only half-joking comment I've often heard from individuals who are involved in caring for the elderly. Yet, as much as Americans plan for their futures earlier in life, few of us dare think about and plan for frailty, which could extend over years or even decades of our lives. *Aging with a Plan* aims to change that.

The book is anchored in both my personal experience and my professional expertise as a professor of law and bioethics at Case Western Reserve University. I am also a member of the Ethics Committee at Cleveland's University Hospitals, which often grapples with difficult treatment decisions for incapacitated elderly persons who do not have other decision makers. My interest in issues of health law, bioethics, and care giving stems in part from a 15-month period in the mid-1990s in which I suffered my own medical crisis and shortly thereafter became a caregiver for my then 65-year-old mother, who underwent extensive treatment for breast cancer.

The first time I thought seriously about my mortality was in the spring of 1994. I awoke in the early morning hours of May 4 to the most severe abdominal pain I had ever experienced. I struggled to think clearly. Was it a stomach flu? Was it menstrual cramps? I got out of bed and walked doubled-over to the bathroom. I took two aspirin, fought my urge to shriek in agony, and tried to find the least uncomfortable position, alternately sitting, lying down, and pacing in my small one-bedroom apartment. I could not believe how piercing and unrelenting the pain was, and nothing would relieve it.

I was 29, single, and had no family in Houston, where I had been living for four years. It turned out that I had a large (eight by five by five inches), borderline malignant ovarian tumor. I underwent major surgery but, to my relief, no chemotherapy or radiation was needed. Once the diagnosis was made, my parents, who lived in Michigan, rushed to Houston and friends remained by my side so that I was rarely left alone until well after my hospitalization. Six weeks after the surgery, at the end of June, I resumed my full-time work schedule. I weighed 98 pounds, having lost 10 pounds, and tired easily, but life slowly returned to normal.

And then came a phone call in the third week of November 1994 that would dramatically change everything once again. My mother, or Eema, as we called her in Hebrew, was diagnosed with breast cancer following suspicious findings on a routine mammogram. She wanted to take advantage of my living in Houston and be seen at the renowned M.D. Anderson Cancer Center. Thus, my parents and three younger sisters made a pilgrimage to Texas, and my one-bedroom apartment turned into Hoffman Family Headquarters.

Eema had a full mastectomy to remove her right breast along with 12 lymph nodes on December 7, 1994. The surgery was successful, but we soon learned that six of the lymph nodes were positive for cancer. She would need both chemotherapy and radiation, with treatment lasting well into the summer.

I don't remember any serious family discussion of next steps. Instead, I remember only Eema's announcement: "I'm going to stay in Houston for all of my treatment. I will live with Sharona, and everyone else can visit when you want to."

I had not contemplated this possibility before, but I did not object. It was reasonable for Eema to want to be treated at a premier oncology center, so I embarked on this journey with her, though not without trepidation.

And thus began what ironically became one of the most wonderful periods of my life. Eema had always been a devoted mother, but I considered her to be more a strict disciplinarian than a friend during my first three decades. By contrast, the nine months I spent with Eema in Houston were a gift that introduced me to a person I had never known before. Eema suddenly blossomed into a gregarious, adventurous, and fun-loving woman who looked and acted decades younger than her 65 years.

We attended numerous lectures and community events. We also frequently went to the theater and took advantage of half-priced tickets that were available one hour before the show began. Eema even developed a surprising interest in eating out, though she had previously always preferred to eat modest meals at home.

I would tease Eema and tell her that she was exhausting me with all this running around. "You're supposed to be sick, and I'm supposed to be having a very boring year, stuck in the apartment taking care of you. Instead, you don't let me stay home at all."

In response she would squeal in delight and acknowledge that she didn't recognize herself. "Who knows what's really in this chemo? It is giving me a complete personality overhaul."

Eema's energy, initiative, and magnetism impressed me to no end. Her caregivers loved her. My friends adored her. Even Freddie, the woman who delivered our mail, was extremely fond of her because Eema made a point of going downstairs to the mailboxes to chat with her as she worked. Freddie asked about Eema whenever she saw me for years thereafter.

Eema completed her eight cycles of chemotherapy and then underwent six weeks of radiation treatment. She left Houston in August 1995 and was cancer free for almost 18 years. She died on May 17, 2013, of what turned out to be pancreatic cancer.

I often think back to the dramatic years of 1994–95. I have been both a patient with a serious illness and a caregiver for a prolonged period of time. I learned firsthand about the triumphs of modern medicine and the challenges and complexities of the health care and insurance industries. I also learned a lot about care giving. I know how important family, friends, and community are in difficult times. And I have an acute awareness of how much time, effort, and money may be required to meet all the needs of a loved one who is very ill.

Eema and I were sustained by the devotion of our friends and by our own close bond. We looked forward to visits, phone calls, and mail, and we made a point of going out and interacting with others as often as possible. The many months we spent together were also a highlight for me because I felt at my most useful, and Eema was generous in expressing her gratitude every day. For others whose health is failing, it is very challenging to maintain robust social lives and a sense of purpose. The importance of social interaction and feeling useful are major themes throughout this book.

My experiences led me to become increasingly interested in medical matters and ultimately to devote my career to health law and bioethics. A decade after graduating from Harvard Law School in 1988, I returned to school to pursue an advanced degree (LL.M) in health law at the University of Houston Law Center and then obtained a faculty position at Case Western Reserve University School of Law, where I serve as codirector of the Law-Medicine Center.

I have written *Aging with a Plan* in order to find answers to the many questions and anxieties that I have about growing old without an obvious source of informal care giving. In 2013, Eema suffered terribly during a 10-day hospitalization before her pancreatic cancer was diagnosed, and we switched her to hospice care for the final two days of her life. But in some ways, she was very fortunate. Once it was clear that Eema's condition was serious, her four daughters dropped everything and rushed to be with her, and we left the hospital only to get a few hours of sleep at night. We also were not shy about pressing doctors and nurses to do everything possible to relieve her pain, and we easily reached consensus about pursuing comfort care when it was clear the end was near. Eema took her last breath while deeply asleep and surrounded by her children.

Thereafter, our father, though he was devastated by the loss of his wife of 54 years, enjoyed the benefits of having four devoted daughters. One of my three sisters resided minutes away and was extremely involved in his care. She visited frequently, filled his pill boxes, and coordinated all of his care. The rest of us, who lived out of state, called multiple times a week and visited as often as we could. When it was clear my father was dying in late 2014, we once again gathered together and held a vigil by his bedside until he took his last breath.

My old age will inevitably be different. My husband, Andy, is seven years older than I, and we have no children and no large, extended family. Moreover, in October 2013, at the age of 55, Andy was diagnosed with Parkinson's disease. Although this illness progresses slowly, it is likely that he will become increasingly disabled in the future and need assistance from paid caregivers, which could deplete our savings. These circumstances worry me. If I reach old age and suffer the inevitable deterioration of my health, will I have a strong support network, as I did when I was sick at 29? In the absence of children, will there be trustworthy people who can regularly help me with medications, transportation, finances, and the like? If I live independently in old age, will I have the fortitude to give up driving when that is prudent or to know when it is time to seek professional care giving or move to a nursing home? And what if I become one of the millions of elderly people who suffer cognitive impairment and dementia? How can I even begin to contemplate that possibility?

Over the years I have learned that many share my anxiety about having to be self-reliant in old age. What can be done? One option is to simply focus on enjoying the present and not "waste time" fretting about potential future misfortunes. But a need to manage and plan is deeply embedded in my nature. Letting the chips fall where they may is not. You can always hope to die in your sleep, but studies estimate that only 7 to 15 percent of elderly people experience sudden death with no prior diagnosis of a potentially fatal illness.[1] Some torments, like the onset of dementia, are currently outside of human control. But other hardships, like social isolation and a lack of purpose, can be overcome or avoided with sufficient effort.

In the spring of 2007, I spent a sabbatical semester at the Centers for Disease Control and Prevention, working on public health emergency preparedness. Although it is certainly possible that any of us will experience a public health emergency such as a flu outbreak or hurricane, it is even more likely that we will live to be elderly. This book, therefore, serves as a guide to old-age preparedness.

A FEW FACTS AND FIGURES

The challenges of aging are of utmost importance to American society and will only grow in significance in the coming years and decades. If you are like me and are hitting the half-century mark, you are among a large wave of people who are changing the age demographics in this country.

According to government statistics, in 2012, 13 percent of the population, or 43 million people, were age 65 and over,[2] up from 3 million in 1900.[3] Those who are 85 years old and older numbered 5.9 million in 2012, compared to just over 100,000 in 1900. Experts predict that by 2050, the 85 and older population will grow to 18 million.[4]

"Baby boomers," defined as those born between 1946 and 1964, began turning 65 in 2011. The 65 and older population is projected to expand to

72 million by 2030 and to represent nearly 20 percent of total U.S. residents. After 2030, the proportion of elderly individuals will stabilize at 20 percent, though their absolute number will continue to grow along with the U.S population.

In 2012, life expectancy in the United States was 76.4 years for males and 81.2 years for women.[5] Life expectancy is an average that varies with age, and thus the outlook is even better for individuals who have already lived to be 65, because they have survived hazards that are typically faced earlier in life, such as during infancy, childhood, and young adulthood.[6] Women who are now 65 can expect to reach age 85 and men age 82, and within this population, over 25 percent will live to be 90 years old or older.[7]

Although many seniors achieve longevity, they do not necessarily do so in good health. In 2009–10, 45 percent of Americans aged 65 and older had been diagnosed with two or more chronic conditions, including, most commonly, hypertension, heart disease, diabetes, cancer, stroke, chronic bronchitis, emphysema, asthma, and kidney disease.[8]

Furthermore, over 5 million Americans suffer from Alzheimer's disease and many others suffer from other forms of dementia. Most of these individuals are 65 and older.[9] Recent research, however, provides some encouraging news concerning dementia. One study found that dementia rates among residents of England and Wales who are 65 and older dropped from 8.3 percent in the early 1990s to 6.2 percent in 2011.[10] Several other studies confirm a decline in the prevalence of dementia.[11] This drop is likely attributable to better education and health, including control of blood pressure and cholesterol[12] through medication and good health habits such as regular exercise and a Mediterranean diet.[13]

Nevertheless, dementia was estimated to cost $214 billion in the United States in 2014.[14] Much of the burden of caring for this population falls on family and friends. According to one source, over 15.5 million Americans provide unpaid care for Alzheimer's disease and other dementia patients, supplying an estimated 17.7 billion hours of care in 2013.[15]

But many individuals lack adequate support systems. Federal government statistics reveal that in 2010, women who were 65 or older were twice as likely to live alone as men in that age group (37 percent versus 19 percent).[16] Overall, 12.1 million seniors live alone, constituting approximately 28 percent of the noninstitutionalized older population.[17] One source estimates that this figure includes at least 25 percent of dementia patients who live in the community.[18]

The Childless

It is particularly notable that a growing segment of the U.S. population remains childless throughout life. As of 2012, according to the Census Bureau, 16.1 percent of women in the age group of 40 to 50 had never given birth.[19] In 1976, the figure was only 10 percent. Experts predict that 22 percent of women born in the years 1956 to 1972 will not have children,[20] and the number of U.S. couples without children is projected to increase by 37 percent by 2025.[21]

In her moving memoir *Blue Nights*, Joan Didion writes about the death of her only daughter less than two years after she lost her husband. In a poignant passage with particular resonance for me, she recounts her efforts to fill out medical forms in physicians' offices:

> Sitting in frigid waiting rooms trying to think of the name and telephone number of the person I want notified in case of emergency.
>
> Whole days now spent on this question. This question with no possible answer: *who do I want notified in case of emergency?*

She could think of no one, and left the space blank on the paper.[22] Many others who lack close relatives must face similar dispiriting moments. A major purpose of this book is to offer resources and recommendations for those who will be aging without nearby family members to whom they can turn for assistance.

WHAT THE BOOK COVERS

Aging with a Plan offers one-stop shopping to those who wish to prepare for their own old age and that of loved ones. I explore a variety of relevant social, legal, financial, and medical issues. I elaborate on the importance of developing a robust social life, intellectual interests, and ways to maintain a sense of purposefulness that will not fade late in life. In the words of a friend who is a geriatric social worker, the key to good aging is to "stay active physically, mentally, and socially."

In general, my guiding question is: What should middle-aged individuals contemplate, study, decide, and do to be as well equipped as possible for their own aging and that of loved ones? Furthermore, at a broader, societal level, what cultural, attitudinal, and legal changes are required to improve the prospects of the elderly, especially those who cannot count on others to care for them? What should baby boomers, with their strong political voice and economic power, be striving and lobbying for?

In brief, I address the following topics in this book's chapters.

I explore some of the costs that individuals may incur after retirement and discuss the importance of retirement savings and of obtaining professional financial advice. I provide guidance as to how to obtain financial counseling and begin a savings program and analyze in detail two particular financial products: long-term care insurance and reverse mortgages.

I describe several types of retirement communities with a special focus on continuing care retirement communities. I argue that seniors should not lightly dismiss the idea of living in a community setting because of the importance of maintaining social interaction and intellectual and civic engagement throughout life.

A major concern for independent seniors without close family members is whether anyone will be available to help coordinate their care, pay bills, and provide the support that others receive from their children and nearby relatives. I explore a variety of emerging options for professional help, namely geriatric care managers, daily money managers, elder law attorneys, professional organizers, and experts who can assist with adapting a home to accommodate disabilities or with preparing it for sale.

I discuss and critique a variety of documents that are essential for the purposes of legal preparedness: durable powers of attorney for health care, living wills, organ donation forms, advance directives for mental health treatment, durable powers of attorney for property and finances, wills, and trusts.

I dedicate a chapter to the fraught issue of driving by the elderly. I examine whether elderly drivers have reason to worry that they are a danger to themselves or others on the road, how state laws handle driver's license renewal in old age, how families can tell whether elderly relatives are at risk of unsafe driving, and how to approach conversations with elderly loved ones regarding this sensitive subject. I also discuss transportation alternatives that are available in some communities and emerging automobile technologies that will enhance seniors' ability to drive safely as they grow older.

I focus on the changing medical needs of people from middle age onward and the importance of obtaining coordinated care, ideally from physicians with geriatric expertise. I also outline strategies for becoming an active, educated member of your own medical team and for building strong support networks in case of illness or disability.

I discuss the long-term care needs of the elderly and the existing options for such care. To this end, I analyze the benefits and shortcomings of nursing homes, assisted living, home care, and adult day services. I also provide guidance to help you do your research and make appropriate choices concerning long-term care.

I analyze end-of-life care and the degree to which you can maintain control over it. I discuss assisted suicide (available in a handful of states), the ability to decline unwanted life-prolonging treatment, "do not resuscitate" orders, palliative care, and hospice programs. Thinking about the end of life might seem like a depressing thing to do, but engaging in soul-searching about our preferences, knowing what choices we'll have, and discussing these matters with loved ones should facilitate end-of-life decision making for ourselves and those in our care.

Since my husband's Parkinson's disease diagnosis, I am more aware than ever before that life is unpredictable and that, in the words of an old adage, sometimes "people make plans and God laughs." The diagnosis came at age 55, when we believed that Andy had many, many years of good health and full strength ahead of him. Parkinson's disease is a degenerative neurologic condition caused by loss of dopamine cells in the brain, and patients often live for decades with it. We simply do not know what the future holds for us in terms of Andy's disease progression, ability to work, care needs, and expenses. At the same time that we must accept considerable uncertainty (a particularly difficult proposition for me), we must also try even harder to put safeguards in place so that our future is as secure as possible in terms of finances and opportunities for social, intellectual, and civic engagement.

Planning ahead can be critical to maintaining a good quality of life in old age even when you suffer health problems, loss of loved ones, and other misfortunes. By contrast, facing a crisis without having thought about potential next steps can be overwhelming. Crisis can come in many forms: sudden illness, death of a spouse, or worsening mental or physical impairments that rob a person of the ability to take care of him- or herself. Without planning ahead, these adversities can leave elderly individuals without any good options, unable to socialize, to remain active and independent, and to enjoy the pleasures that make life worth living.

Planning for old age entails not only taking concrete steps, such as writing a will and an advance directive, but also learning about the problems that the elderly encounter, such as obstacles to effective medical care and driving challenges. Learning about these matters will not only help you think through how you might address them when your time comes, but will also empower you to help aging loved ones in the more immediate future.

With adequate planning, the long-term impact of hardships can be diminished. Furthermore, planning ahead can prevent the loss of autonomy that so many seniors fear. For example, having a trusted substitute decision maker can alleviate anxiety about what financial and medical decisions will be made for you if you lose decision-making capacity. Likewise, living in a high-quality retirement community can be a solution to the problems of social isolation and inactivity in old age.

In short, the book strives to develop sound approaches to building sustainable social, medical, and financial support mechanisms that can increase the likelihood of a good quality of life throughout the aging process. In other words, I aim to develop a plan that will be useful to me and, more important, to you.

1

Money Matters: Retirement Expenses, Savings, and Fiscal Decision Making

Many decisions about retirement, living environment, health care, and other matters related to aging depend at least in part on finances. Money may not buy happiness, but being financially comfortable can make it easier to live a satisfying and enjoyable life after retirement. Your ability to follow several (though certainly not all) of the recommendations outlined in this book will depend on having adequate resources, and, therefore, I address money matters upfront.

Baby boomers will become eligible for full social security benefits at age 66 if born before 1960 or at age 67 if born in 1960 or later.[1] Thus, millions of Americans could live for two or more decades after retirement. With what money will they support themselves? This chapter will discuss what can be done in middle age to maximize the possibility of having a financially comfortable older age.

ARE AMERICANS SAVING ENOUGH?

I have heard friends joke that "My kids are my retirement plan." In reality, however, contemporary parents more often find themselves supporting adult children than being supported by them. According to the Census Bureau, in 2012, 13.6 percent of 25- to 34-year-old Americans lived with their parents.[2] In addition, 10 percent of grandparents have a grandchild living with them.[3]

Furthermore, a national Pew Research Center survey found that 48 percent of adults ages 40 to 59 provided at least one child with financial support in 2012, and 27 percent were the primary source of support. By contrast, only 21 percent of middle-aged adults provided financial support to parents who were 65 or older that same year.[4]

Many commentators bemoan the fact that most Americans' retirement savings are sorely inadequate. The Employee Benefits Research Institute found that in 2012,[5] 60 percent of workers had household savings and investments that totaled less than $25,000, exclusive of the value of their primary homes and defined benefits plans.* A different source reports that four of five Americans are saving less than 10 percent of their incomes for retirement,[6] and the Social Security Administration estimates that 34 percent of the workforce has no savings designated for retirement.[7] This is not to say that workers should be blamed for their savings shortfall. In many cases it is the inevitable result of low earnings and the high price of essentials such as housing, higher education, and health care and not a consequence of individuals' choices to spend on luxury items today rather than save for tomorrow.

SENIORS' MEDICAL EXPENSES

Financial resources make it possible to enjoy leisure activities in old age. But even more important, they are essential to obtaining proper medical care after retirement. Even retirees who live modestly can expect to have considerable expenses because of uncovered health care costs. An Urban Institute study published in 2010[8] predicted that seniors' median out-of-pocket annual expenditures for medical care would be $3,284 in 2020 and $6,214 in 2040.† These estimates do not include long-term care costs.

Some services needed by seniors are rarely covered by insurance—hearing aids, for example. Unfortunately, these devices cost $3,000 to $7,000, a price that is daunting or completely unaffordable for all too many retirees.[9] Even more significantly, the elderly generally have to pay out of pocket for

---

*Defined benefit plans promise a specified monthly payment after retirement, consisting of either a particular dollar amount or payment based on a formula that takes into account factors such as the employee's salary and service. By contrast, defined contribution plans do not promise specific payments. Rather, these plans allow the employer, employee, or both to contribute to the employee's account, and payment after retirement depends on the amount accumulated. Examples of defined contribution plans are 401(k) and 403(b) plans. "Retirement Plans, Benefits & Savings, Types of Plans," United States Department of Labor, accessed October 17, 2014, http://www.dol.gov/dol/topic /retirement/typesofplans.htm.

†At the 75th percentile, the annual estimates were: $3,934 in 2010; $4,959 in 2020; $6,855 in 2030; and $9,455 in 2040. These estimates are in constant 2008 dollars.

in-home care, assisted living, and often nursing home care, which costs tens of thousands of dollars per year.

A study published in 2012 investigated patients' out-of-pocket medical expenditures during the final five years of life. It concluded that average total spending for those last five years was $38,688 for individuals. Furthermore, 43 percent of subjects incurred costs that exceeded their assets (excluding their homes).[10]

How much money might you need to meet your medical costs after retirement? Fidelity Investments estimates that a 65-year-old couple will need $240,000 to cover future medical expenses, such as deductibles, copayments, and the many costs that Medicare does not cover.[11] This figure does not include the very high price of long-term care. As discussed in Chapter 7, on average, nursing homes cost approximately $85,000 per year for a private room and $75,000 for a semiprivate room, the base rate for a one-bedroom apartment in an assisted living facility is approximately $42,000, and home care agencies charge around $19 per hour for aides. If an elderly individual needs to reside in a facility or receive round-the-clock care at home, the costs can grow to be astronomical.

A study published in 2013 in the *American Journal of Law and Medicine* asked 1,700 individuals to estimate their postretirement out-of-pocket expenditures for health care. The authors found that over 50 percent of respondents underestimated the costs projected by experts. Furthermore, respondents failed to understand that spending levels are uncertain and can vary because of changes in a patient's health status, health care pricing, and government policies.[12] Likewise, a 2013 Pew survey found that a majority of Americans are optimistic about their financial prospects in retirement, with 63 percent answering that they are "very" or "somewhat" confident that they will have an adequate standard of living when they are old.[13]

However, reality may be quite different for many. It is safe to assume that an alarming number of retirees will not be able to live comfortably, much less luxuriously, in old age. Those who are parents should be aware that their lack of savings could generate considerable financial obligations for their children. For example, in 2012, a Pennsylvania court held that a son was required to pay a $92,943 bill for his mother's nursing home care following a car accident.[14] Twenty-nine states have filial support laws that require adult children to support impoverished parents. The statutes have rarely been enforced, but long-term care institutions may choose to rely upon them as a collection tool.[15]

RETIREMENT SAVINGS AND PROFESSIONAL FINANCIAL ADVICE

It may seem obvious that money is essential to a comfortable aging process, especially if you will age without many close family members nearby who can provide unpaid assistance. However, the statistics above indicate that many may not have internalized this message, and, according to the Employee Benefits Research Institute, 56 percent of workers report that they and their spouses have not even attempted to calculate how much money they would need for retirement.[16] Consequently, the desirability of devising a financial plan bears mentioning.

As a first step, those whose employers offer a defined contribution plan such as a 401(k) should be sure to enroll. Saving through these plans is rewarded with tax benefits because money is taken out of paychecks before taxes. As a simple example, if you are taxed at a 25 percent rate, you receive only $75 for every $100 of your salary. However, if you designate $100 for your 401(k) account, the entire amount is invested because the 25 percent tax is not collected. Moreover, employers often match at least a percentage of contributions, thus adding considerably to workers' retirement savings. Yet, 20 to 30 percent of eligible workers fail to join available 401(k) plans.[17]

If your employer offers life insurance and disability insurance at little to no cost, you should also be sure to sign up for these benefits. Life insurance will provide your named beneficiary or beneficiaries with a sum of money upon your death, which they can use however they see fit, including to pay for your funeral. Disability insurance will pay all or part of your salary if you become unable to work because of a disability.

Life insurance is particularly valuable for individuals of modest means whose families may not have funds to pay for burial expenses. If it is possible that this will be true of your family, you should purchase a policy even if it is not available through your employer.

You can also speak to your bank about opening a traditional individual retirement account (IRA) or a Roth IRA. Contributions to a Roth IRA are limited to $5,500 (or $6,500 for those 50 and over), and the money is tax exempt when it is withdrawn.[18]

In addition, deferring retirement for a few years will not only enable you to earn extra income, but will also raise the amount of your social security payments. The Social Security Administration offers delayed retirement credits to eligible individuals. As the federal regulations explain: "[y]ou may earn a credit for each month during the period beginning with the month you attain full retirement age (as defined in §404.409) and ending with the month you attain age 70."[19] Full retirement age ranges from 65 for those born before 1938 to 67 for those born in 1960 or thereafter.[20]

Experts advise that you save for retirement even if you have young children and simultaneously need to save for their college educations. College loans are widely available, but similar borrowing programs do not exist for retirement. And failing to save for retirement may well mean that you will become a burden to your children later on.[21]

Even small savings can accrue to meaningful sums over the years. For example, saving just $1 a day during a single year for a total of $365 would yield $1,577.50 after 30 years assuming a 5 percent interest rate. An individual who continuously saves $250 each month in an account with an interest rate of just 1 percent would have $15,637.57 after 5 years of maintaining this fiscal habit.[22]

Those with more financial flexibility should engage in thoughtful retirement planning. There is no magic formula to calculate how much one should save for retirement.[23] The answer depends largely on one's preferred lifestyle, reasonably anticipated earnings from investments and pension plans, and expected number of years without work. Various retirement calculators on the Internet can serve as a starting point for computing a ballpark amount of savings that you should have prior to retirement. For example, Moneychimp's "Simple Retirement Calculator" readily computes an annual retirement income based on three questions: (1) current principal; (2) preretirement annual additions, years to grow, and growth rate; and (3) postretirement years to pay out and growth rate.[24] A more sophisticated tool called "Choose to Save" asks users 16 questions. Be aware that some of the queries, such as "expected age at death" and "inflation assumption," are quite speculative and ask for predictions of the unpredictable.[25]

Relying on the Internet should not be the final step. Those who are concerned about their financial futures should consult trustworthy financial professionals at least periodically. Many workplaces offer employees opportunities to speak with retirement experts at no cost.

Low income earners may also be able to obtain financial planning advice at no charge from professional volunteers. For example most chapters of the Financial Planning Association (FPA) offer free help to underserved populations,[26] and you can search on the Internet for an FPA chapter in your state and obtain contact information for pro bono services.[27] In addition, a wealth of information can be found on a website called Wife.org, run by a nonprofit organization that is "dedicated to providing an unbiased, financial education to women in their quest for financial independence."[28] Of course, you do not have to be a woman to read the information on this website!

If you will be hiring a financial adviser at your own expense, you should seek recommendations from knowledgeable acquaintances. You should also carefully interview potential advisers to determine their level of experience, fee structure, and whether they are committed to selling particular financial products to their clients because their companies require them to do so. You should look for a certified financial planner rather than an individual with no certification. You will also want to know if the individual charges a flat fee or an hourly fee or is compensated by commission only. Flat fees can take the form of a particular sum, such as $1,500, or a percentage of your assets, typically 1 percent. Paying a fee equivalent to 1 percent of your assets may be daunting if you are fairly well off. On the other hand, advisers working on commission might be motivated to recommend that you make frequent changes that will yield a commission for them or that you purchase particular assets that will put more money in their pockets. You may want to ask candidates for the names of a couple of clients whom you can call as references to determine their level of satisfaction.[29]

Financial advisers can help clients develop savings plans, follow them, and diversify their portfolios to provide some degree of protection against market vicissitudes. Competent advisers will formulate investment strategies based on how much financial risk their clients want to tolerate and what the clients' investment objectives are, as well as general rules of thumb. A particularly important decision is that of asset allocation, that is, choosing the appropriate combination of stocks, bonds, and possibly other assets (e.g., real estate).[30] In a strong stock market, stocks can be very lucrative, but they can also quickly plummet in value when the market falls. By contrast, bonds pay a fixed interest rate for a designated period of time, though the interest rate often provides less income than stocks with high dividends.

Some experts advise that the percentage of stocks in an individual's portfolio should be determined roughly by subtracting the investor's age from 100, with the remainder allocated to bonds, or, alternatively, that the percentage of money in bonds should be derived by multiplying the investor's age by 80 percent. Under the first formula, a 65-year-old should have 65 percent of her money in bonds and 35 percent in stocks; under the second, less conservative formula, she should have only 52 percent in bonds and 48 percent in stocks.[31] To maintain the preferred asset allocation over time, the investor will periodically need to adjust the distribution of her money as earnings vary in the different asset categories.[32] Asset diversification lowers the risk of loss because if one sector, such as the stock market, has a downturn, the investor will still have a significant portion of her assets in other sectors that are not experiencing similar weakness.

Even those who are self-motivated to save will benefit from professional support. In early 2013, an ordinary savings or money market account paid an interest rate of 0.03 percent. How can you build meaningful savings with an essentially nonexistent growth rate? Today's economy requires more sophisticated investment choices than simply putting your money in a bank's savings account.

It is difficult, even for an experienced investor, to avoid having a few investment portfolio failures. To maintain a sense of perspective, develop realistic expectations and know what questions to ask. It is prudent to remain updated about the market and to engage in some degree of self-education. Nevertheless, for me, at least, peace of mind depends on having a professional expert look after my savings.

Financial planning advice may become increasingly affordable and accessible if it is available through the Internet. Start-up companies such as

LearnVest are developing products that enable consumers to obtain planning services through a website at relatively modest fees.[33]

Retiring with adequate savings will not guarantee a healthy and fulfilling aging experience because illness and misfortune can intervene regardless of the size of one's bank account. However, the value of a comfortable monthly income in retirement cannot be ignored. It will enable seniors to move to retirement communities (discussed in the next chapter) if they wish to do so, pursue travel and other pleasures, and obtain the best available medical and personal care when necessary.

I now turn to two financial products that you may consider in planning your fiscal future: long-term care insurance and reverse mortgages. In each case, there are clear potential benefits but also significant pitfalls.

LONG-TERM CARE INSURANCE

When I first began researching long-term care insurance, I thought purchasing such insurance would be an easy call. I am generally risk-averse, and in the absence of children who could become unpaid caregivers, obtaining a policy would surely be prudent. It turns out that, as in the case of so many other matters related to elder care, there is no clear and certain answer to the question of whether you should buy long-term care insurance.

Long-term care costs, estimated as between $211 and $306 billion annually,[34] represent approximately 9 percent of health care expenditures in the United States. These expenses are covered largely by public sources, with Medicare paying 24 percent and Medicaid 43 percent. The remainder is generally paid by individuals out of pocket. Long-term care insurance policies are responsible for a mere 4 to 7 percent of payments.[35]

Only about 14 percent of Americans who are 60 or older have long-term care insurance policies.[36] This low number may be explained by the fact that long-term care insurance is expensive compared to its benefits.

Long-term care insurance policies cover all or some of the following services: nursing home stays, assisted living, adult day care, and home care. Contracts specify the conditions under which coverage is triggered. Typically, coverage becomes available when the policyholder needs significant assistance with a minimum of two activities of daily living (e.g., bathing and dressing) because of physical limitations that are expected to last at least 90 days or because of severe cognitive impairment. Before this point of advanced disability, the insurer will not reimburse customers for expenses even if they obtain help from professional caregivers. A majority of policies are sold individually to customers, but a growing number of employers are offering group plans, though they do not subsidize them.[37]

Typical policies have a variety of limitations that should give you pause. Most policies require high premiums and exclude coverage for an initial period of time, generally ranging from the first 30 to 90 days of long-term care. Because the median nursing home stay is three months for men and eight months for women, that exclusion may prevent a large number of policyholders from obtaining any reimbursement for nursing home costs.[38] Most policies restrict benefits to no more than one to eight years, and only about one-quarter allow for benefits of unlimited duration. In addition, most policies limit benefits to a maximum dollar amount per day. In 2005, the average daily maximum for nursing home payments from policies was $142, while the average daily cost of such care in 2008 was $200. If the designated top payment amount is fixed and a purchaser uses benefits decades after obtaining her policy, she may find that costs have risen significantly. Therefore, the policy will cover her for a smaller percentage of care expenditures than anticipated. Even if benefits grow over time under policy terms, the increases often do not fully adjust for inflation.[39]

What premiums can consumers expect to pay? As indicated in the table on page 9, according to the National Association of Insurance Commissioners, premiums vary widely, and many purchasers pay thousands of dollars per year.[40] In light of the policies' high premiums and benefit restrictions, the typical policyholder can expect to receive only 68 cents in benefits for every dollar paid in premiums,* according to experts.[41]

Consumers often allow their policies to lapse because of the high costs of premiums and the uncertainty of deriving significant future benefits. Individuals who become financially stressed may see the considerable expense of the annual premium as one they can easily eliminate without suffering any immediate adversity. According to one source, an average of 5 percent of policies lapse per year. If you let your policy lapse, you get no return whatsoever on your investment of thousands upon thousands of premium dollars paid before you canceled the policy.[42] Some insurers offer nonforfeiture benefits, which allow you to get some value for your policy if you stop paying premiums, but these benefits add significantly to your costs.[43]

Medicaid is yet another factor that complicates the decision of whether to buy a long-term care insurance policy. Individuals with few financial resources can obtain Medicaid coverage for nursing home care once they spend down their assets. Detailed guidelines determine Medicaid eligibility, as discussed at greater length in Chapter 7. Typically, single people can keep their home, personal effects, and vehicle but must have no more than

---

*For an accurate estimate, the calculation must take into account the present discounted values of premiums and benefits. The idea is that money that you have at present is worth more than money you will obtain in the future because it can earn interest or be invested in the interim.

Average Annual Premium for Basic Long-Term Insurance $200 Daily Benefit*

Age When Bought	With Inflation Protection 5% Compounded Per Year		
	4 Years of Benefits	*6 Years of Benefits*	*Lifetime Benefits*
50	$4,349	$5,083	$7,347
60	$5,331	$6,269	$8,927
70	$9,206	$10,549	$15,070
75	$13,500	$15,157	$20,930
	With No Inflation Protection—Benefit Stays at $200 Per Day		
	4 Years of Benefits	*6 Years of Benefits*	*Lifetime Benefits*
50	$1,294	$1,514	$1,997
60	$2,057	$2,426	$3,307
70	$4,914	$5,834	$7,777
75	$8,146	$8,291	$12,337

*Reprinted by permission from National Association of Insurance Commissioners, *Buyer's Guide to Long-Term Care Insurance* (Kansas City, MO: National Association of Insurance Commissioners 2013), 33.

$2,000 in "countable resources" (cash, financial accounts, stocks, bonds, available assets in trust).[44] Long-term care insurance could in fact constitute a barrier to Medicaid coverage if it is considered an asset that disqualifies you from Medicaid eligibility.[45] Moreover, even for those who qualify for benefits, Medicaid will pay for care only after long-term care insurance payments have been exhausted. Therefore, you might find that you spent tens of thousands of dollars on long-term care insurance but still end up impoverished and on Medicaid. The only party that actually benefits in this scenario is Medicaid, which has to pay less for your long-term care. Therefore, owning policies is of no advantage to anyone who would otherwise become Medicaid eligible.[46]

By contrast, people with significant income and assets may be wiser to save and invest the money that would otherwise be spent on premiums. Wealthy individuals can afford to take the gamble. If long-term care is needed, you can pay for it even without an insurance policy, and if no long-term care is ever needed, you will have saved the considerable expenditure of paying for a policy of which you will never take advantage.

Various government interventions could make long-term care insurance more appealing in the future. Tax incentives could partially subsidize the cost of policies. Some states have instituted partnership programs that allow individuals who purchase qualifying long-term care insurance plans to retain a designated amount of assets and still qualify for Medicaid.[47] The

Community Living Assistance Services and Supports (CLASS) Act, which was part of President Barack Obama's Patient Protection and Affordable Care Act of 2010, would have enabled the federal government to sell private long-term care insurance policies directly to the public. This program, however, was abandoned in 2011 because it was deemed not to be financially viable.[48] Although it is unlikely that federal and state governments will provide significant support for long-term care insurance purchases in the near future, it is possible that such proposals will be revived later on as the population continues to age.[49]

So, should you buy long-term care insurance? On the one hand, premium payments run in the thousands of dollars annually and will likely rise in the future.[50] Whether or not you will ever derive any plan benefits is uncertain because your long-term care needs will be unpredictable at the time of purchase. Because policies are often purchased decades before benefits are needed, another small risk is that your insurer will become insolvent before you require long-term care, so your policy won't be honored. On the other hand, research suggests that 5 percent of individuals who are 65 and older incur long-term care costs in excess of $250,000, and for such patients, insurance might be invaluable. Jesse Slome, executive director of the American Association for Long-Term Care Insurance, stated that "insurers paid some $6.6 billion in benefits to roughly 200,000 individuals" in 2011.[51] There is simply no way to predict what your needs will be at the end of life.

Financial advisers' recommendations as to who should buy long-term care insurance vary. According to the Society of Actuaries, the purchase may be unwise for (1) those with savings of less than $200,000 to 250,000* and (2) those with assets greater than $2 million.[52] Another commentator, Prescott Cole, a senior staff attorney at California Advocates for Nursing Home Reform, asserts that for "those with little wealth, a policy will never be suitable" because of the existence of Medicaid. He adds that people whose annual income is $250,000 or more with "substantial savings" also should not purchase long-term care insurance.[53]

For those of us in the middle, the question is more difficult. Insurers incentivize consumers to make the decision earlier rather than later in life by offering lower premiums for younger purchasers and establishing strict health-based eligibility rules. For example, those with memory loss, mobility limitations, a stroke history, or even mild osteoporosis may be screened out by insurers and deemed ineligible for coverage.[54] On average, people buy policies in their late fifties or early sixties.

---

*A different source states that the figure is $100,000 excluding the home. Steve Weisman, *A Guide to Elder Planning: Everything You Need to Know to Protect Yourself Legally and Financially* (Upper Saddle River, NJ: Prentice Hall, 2004), 153.

My husband became ineligible for long-term care insurance when he received his Parkinson's disease diagnosis at age 55, even though medications and exercise may enable him to continue taking care of himself without paid assistance for several decades. The fact that you could at any time suddenly be disqualified by a diagnosis is the strongest argument for purchasing a policy at a younger rather than older age. Otherwise, you take the risk that you will come to want such a policy but not be able to find an insurer who is willing to sell it to you.

Nevertheless, our financial advisers have urged me not to buy a policy for myself at this time because I am only 50. As much as I like to plan ahead, I have decided to heed their advice and put off this particular decision.

Two new insurance products are also worth considering. Some insurers are offering hybrid long-term care policies in which either life insurance or an annuity is bundled with long-term care coverage. Thus, a savings and investment component is added to insurance.[55] One challenge posed by life insurance hybrids and annuity hybrids is that they generally require very large initial premium payments, such as $50,000.[56] Nevertheless, those with financial means would be prudent to investigate these options.

REVERSE MORTGAGES

Reverse mortgages are heavily advertised on television by celebrities such as Henry Winkler and Fred Thompson. As tempting as these ads make reverse mortgages sound, they too require careful consideration and are not a wise choice for many consumers.

Reverse mortgages are loans that allow borrowers who are at least 62 years old to convert part of the equity in their home into cash, so long as the home is their primary place of residence. Retirees who are homeowners but have limited incomes may rely on these loans to cover basic living expenses and to pay health care costs, though proceeds can be used for any purpose.

The term "reverse mortgage" is used to describe these loans because instead of making monthly payments to a bank, as in the case of traditional mortgages, borrowers receive payments from lenders. Those who obtain reverse mortgages are not required to pay back their loans until the home is sold or otherwise vacated, for example, upon moving to a nursing home or upon death. You need only continue to pay property taxes, homeowners insurance, and condominium fees, if applicable, and to maintain the home in good repair.[57]

So far, so good. However, reverse mortgages come with significant draw-backs. Borrowers incur substantial upfront fees, including mortgage insurance premiums, loan origination fees, and closing costs, as well as ongoing fees such as high interest rates and service fees. *Forbes* has called reverse mortgages "one of the most expensive forms of credit you can get." Also, because the loan must be paid off upon death, heirs may be left with little to inherit.[58] Furthermore, if the reason for leaving the home is a move to a long-term care facility, the loan will become due at the same time that you must begin paying the very high cost of institutional care. Worse yet, a surviving spouse or partner whose name is not on the loan will face foreclosure if he or she cannot pay off the reverse mortgage after the homeowner's death. Foreclosure can also occur if the borrower fails to pay property taxes or homeowners' insurance or does not maintain the home in acceptable condition. Finally, those who choose a lump sum payment and obtain a reverse mortgage in their sixties may exhaust the money long before they need it most.

In some circumstances, reverse mortgages will serve borrowers well as a way to stay in a beloved home and pay living expenses. However, financial advisers often consider reverse mortgages to be a choice of last resort, and seniors should not make the decision to obtain such a loan lightly.

FINANCIAL PREPAREDNESS CHECKLIST

- Save as much as possible for retirement. Do not pass up an opportunity to participate in a 401(k) plan. Recognize that even small amounts of savings can add up over the years.
- Seek professional financial advice. You may be able to obtain advice at no cost through your employer or volunteers in your community. If you hire an adviser, research the candidates' credentials, experience, reputation, and fee structure carefully.
- Do not rush to buy long-term care insurance. Seek a financial adviser's guidance and think carefully about whether this is a wise purchase for you. Consider the option of life insurance or annuity hybrids if you can afford the initial premium payments.
- Understand the limitations and potential pitfalls of reverse mortgages and consider other alternatives before opting for this financial product for yourself or your loved ones.

2

The Benefits of Community Living

One of my relatives, whom I will call Ruth, is a 91-year-old woman who has been widowed for decades and lives alone in the house she has owned for over 50 years. For most of her life, Ruth enjoyed the company of many family members who lived nearby, but she has outlived almost all of them, and now a niece and a neighbor are the only people who visit her regularly. She enjoys restaurants, antique shows, and movies, but she is not comfortable going to these alone. Ruth still drives, and her mental faculties are strong, but she suffers from debilitating back pain and finds it increasingly difficult to manage on her own. Ruth's two children live in a distant state. Although for many years they have encouraged her to move, she resisted doing so while she was content with the life she had, and now she feels it is too late for her to set up an independent life in a new city. In many ways, Ruth is among the lucky because she was able to thrive independently until she was in her nineties. However, now she finds it more and more challenging to maintain her autonomy and avoid social isolation.

The options that come to mind for Ruth are nursing homes, assisted living facilities, and home care, all of which Ruth adamantly rejects. She refuses to enter an institutional setting and does not trust any stranger to provide assistance in her home while she is there alone. She also wants to leave her money to her children rather than spend it on expensive care for herself. The fierce independence and self-sufficiency that served Ruth so well during her first nine decades may be backfiring at this point.

One reason for Ruth's difficult circumstances is that she failed to formulate a plan for her old age. She would immediately change the subject if anyone began a conversation about her future, and she apparently did not turn the matter over in her own mind.

Many Americans, like Ruth, value their autonomy and cling to the hope of remaining in their own homes to the end of their days. A move to a residential setting that is especially designed for seniors may be perceived not only as costly, but also as an admission of defeat, an acknowledgment of loss of vigor and dependency.

Yet, it is unwise to dismiss lightly the idea of living in a community setting. Retirement communities of all types offer the benefits of social interaction and often intellectual and civic engagement through a variety of planned activities and opportunities. Thus, middle-aged individuals who are beginning to plan for their later years or are contemplating options for parents who are finding it difficult to manage in large homes should carefully consider retirement communities.

When my parents were in their mid- to late seventies, they realized that they could no longer safely climb stairs multiple times a day and needed to move out of their large, two-story home. However, our family never contemplated a retirement community and never initiated a conversation about it. Instead, my parents moved into a large condominium with rooms that were all on one floor and ample storage space in the basement that enabled them to keep most of their belongings and avoid the arduous task of culling through them. But this may have been a mistake. My parents became increasingly homebound and socialized less as they grew more frail. Later, as a widower, my father had even fewer opportunities to interact with his contemporaries and was quite lonely, a problem that might have been less pronounced had he lived in a retirement community.

THE IMPORTANCE OF SOCIAL INTERACTION AND FEELING USEFUL

I cannot emphasize enough how important it is to maintain social contacts and a sense of usefulness throughout life. In the words of Epicurus, "Of all the things that wisdom provides for living one's entire life in happiness, the greatest by far is the possession of friendship." In the words of Gretchen Rubin, a contemporary writer, "You need close long-term relationships, you need to be able to confide in others, you need to belong."[1]

Experts have determined that successful social integration is of great importance in the later decades of life.[2] Researchers are learning that social interaction has a significant impact on the health, welfare, and longevity of older adults. Loneliness has been found to be associated with a decline in functioning and death in individuals over 60.[3] For example, loneliness can have an adverse effect on cardiovascular health.[4] It has also been found to cause elevated blood pressure and hormone levels and less sleep.[5] On the other hand, social integration can delay memory decline and preserve cognitive function in seniors.[6] It can also lead to more positive disease outcomes and lengthen life.[7] This is true both nationally and internationally. A study involving over 3,000 Japanese seniors found that activities with family members and friends and a sense of belonging to a neighborhood are "significant predictors of 5-year survival among the seniors."[8] Similarly, a study of 300 elderly individuals in India confirmed that strong social support promotes successful aging in older adults and enhances their sense of control over their lives.[9] Deep friendships that provide people with a sense of self-worth and of being loved may be even more important than family relationships that are obligatory.[10]

Social contact goes hand in hand with feeling useful to others, which is equally important to most people's welfare. An extensive 2009 study published in the *Journal of Aging and Health* concluded that a persistently low perception of usefulness was associated with a shorter lifespan and a reduced sense of well-being, while elderly people with a high perception of social usefulness had better social and health outcomes.[11] Those who are retired and have few family obligations may suffer from "rolelessness" and need to find meaningful activities that enable them to maintain their identity as valued members of society.[12] For example, seniors who volunteered to help students in at-risk public schools scored better than others on tests measuring their health and happiness status.[13]

The importance of meaning and purposefulness does not escape older Americans. The MacArthur Foundation's Study of Successful Aging found that approximately 80 percent of respondents agree with the statement, "Life is not worth living if one cannot contribute to the well-being of others."[14] Dr. George E. Vaillant, who led a Harvard Medical School study of hundreds of individuals with diverse backgrounds, concluded the following in his book *Aging Well*:

> Play, create, learn new things and, most especially, make new friends. Do that and getting out of bed in the morning will seem a joy—even if you are no longer "important," even if your joints ache, and even if you no longer enjoy free access to the office Xerox machine.[15]

Planning for old age, therefore, should include planning to be socially engaged and active. Nurturing friendships and close ties to relatives is beneficial not only for the present but also for the future. The same is true for developing interests, hobbies, and volunteer work. Before retirement, it may often seem that you have little to no time for such pursuits, but engaging in them is worthwhile and necessary, if only as an investment for the future. After retirement, living in a good retirement community can be the key to a happy, social, and fulfilling life.

THE MANY FORMS OF RETIREMENT COMMUNITIES

Retirement communities come in many forms and range widely in cost and structure. A variety of alternatives are worth considering.

Independent Living or 55-Plus Communities

Independent living communities (also known as planned retirement communities) are available in many cities and have amenities that foster social and intellectual engagement. They often offer community centers, activities, meals in a residents' dining hall, transportation services, and more. Some are called "over 55 communities" or "55-plus communities."[16] Retirees may own units or rent apartments, and generally, at least one resident must be 55 or older.

These communities do not offer medical or personal care services. However, they are frequently located near major medical and shopping centers and close to religious and cultural facilities. They have safety features such as guards and emergency buttons, and management handles all repairs. Planned retirement communities market themselves as providing independent seniors with security, convenience, and freedom from the burdens of home maintenance. Some also create a resort-like environment, emphasizing leisure and recreation. Websites such as SeniorHomes.com or A Place for Mom.com can facilitate searches for retirement communities.

Some of my friends whose parents moved to retirement communities in their eighties have reported that their parents were unhappy, especially if they selected the community simply based on its proximity to their children. They found themselves among people who "are not like them," were served food in the dining room that was unpalatable, and were unprepared to meet the challenges of adjusting to a new environment.

But this does not have to be so. A move to a retirement community could be something to which we look forward. If it is financially feasible, people should move while they are still healthy enough to make friends and become active members of the community. Rather than being forced by frailty to move to the facility that is closest to children or siblings, retirees could research a variety of choices and select one that is truly a good fit. Under these more positive circumstances, seniors will hopefully find that friendships come easily because everyone is at the same stage in life and because those who opt for a particular community presumably share common preferences.

An added advantage of moving to a retirement community is that doing so enables seniors to leave homes that are now too large to take care of, have stairs that create a risk of falling, have icy driveways or sidewalks in the winter, or feature other hazards. Housing that is designed specifically for seniors may offer much safer and easier living environments.

Yet another benefit is that moving to a one- or two-bedroom apartment in an independent living community will require most seniors to downsize. Seniors who remain in their large homes rarely cull through their possessions and thoughtfully decide what is essential to keep and to whom the rest should be distributed. This process is often rushed through only when an elderly person is forced to move to an institutional care setting or after death and can cause significant family conflict. Downsizing on their own terms can save elderly people and their families much heartache later on.

Naturally Occurring Retirement Communities and Village Networks

Seniors who seek a community environment are not limited to planned retirement communities. Instead, they may create retirement communities for themselves in their existing homes or in apartment buildings, condominiums, or townhomes to which they move after retirement. Such arrangements have been termed "elder/senior cohousing" or "naturally occurring retirement communities" (NORCs).[17] Those living in a self-created retirement community can check on one another, share caregivers and drivers in order to reduce costs, and carpool together. They can also socialize frequently and participate together in volunteer work, continuing education, and cultural programs.

This approach worked well for my two elderly relatives, Nettie and Mae, who lived to be 96 and 104, respectively. They spent several decades in an apartment complex in Cleveland that catered largely to seniors. Rent was reasonable, and a number of programs were offered each month in a community room, including bingo games and speakers. In addition, a van provided transportation to local destinations for a fee. Nettie and Mae lived in separate apartments "so they would continue to get along well," but they sustained each other through joint activities, daily visits, and many meals together.

Some NORCs have evolved to resemble more formal retirement communities because they are run by professionals and receive financial support from outside sources, which enables residents to benefit from a variety of services. While seniors age in place and do not move to a new home, they can enjoy free or heavily discounted social programs and outings, home delivered meals, assessments of their care needs, yard work and chore services, exercise and preventive health programs, caregiver support groups, classes, and more. For example, a NORC in Toco Hills, an Atlanta suburb, offers seniors a large number of benefits and receives funding through the Jewish Federation and several grants.[18]

Closely related are "village networks," the first of which was Beacon Hill Village in Boston, launched in 2002. Villages are created by residents in particular communities who form nonprofit organizations providing "concierge services," including transportation, home care, house maintenance, and care-management services. They are consumer-driven, membership-based organizations designed, constructed, and governed by those who use them. Members typically pay $500 to $1,000 per person or household per year (with discounts available to those who cannot afford the fee), which covers basic transportation services and regular social events, and other services can be added for a fee. Village networks publish newsletters, host parties, and facilitate further social activities. They are funded through membership dues and donations.[19]

Shared Housing Services

Baby boomers and retirees who are interested in shared housing but find it difficult to identify appropriate housemates might turn to "matchmaking" services. These are available through online vendors as well as through workshops and meetings that take place in local communities. For example, two well-known providers are the National Shared Housing Resource Center and the Golden Girls Network, which serves women only.[20] Financial pressures, a desire for close social ties, and concern about aging alone may all induce individuals (most commonly women) to seek home-sharing living arrangements. You might want a housemate to move into a home you already own or you might want to purchase a new home that is a better fit for elderly people and have one or more co-owners. Entrepreneurs are offering not only matchmaking services but also house-sharing coaching. Coaches counsel clients about financial arrangements, establishing house rules, allocating space, and attending to other logistics.[21]

Senior Centers

Senior centers are not a form of retirement community, but they can provide social and intellectual enrichment and other forms of support for seniors who are living independently or in informal retirement communities. Approximately 11,000 senior centers serve 1 million older Americans. Senior centers offer meals and nutritional programs; fitness and wellness classes; transportation services; counseling regarding public benefits and employment matters; volunteer opportunities; and social, recreational, educational, and arts activities. According to the National Council on Aging (NCOA), the average age of participants is 75, about 70 percent are women, and half live alone. Senior centers receive funding from federal, state, and local government entities but also depend on grants, private donations, and modest fees charged for some activities. The NCOA states enthusiastically that senior center participants "can learn to manage and delay the onset of chronic disease and experience measurable improvements in their physical, social, spiritual, emotional, mental, and economic well-being."[22] You can do a simple Google search for "senior centers in [your city]" in order to locate those that are nearest to you.

Meals on Wheels

Meals on Wheels programs can provide additional support for seniors who are not living in retirement communities with dining services, especially if they are economically disadvantaged. Approximately 5,000 local Senior Nutrition Programs in the United States provide over one million meals to seniors in need each day. Some operate at senior centers; some deliver meals directly to seniors who are homebound and have low incomes; and many programs do both. Programs may ask for modest contributions ($2 or so) or provide food at no cost.[23] Home delivered meals have been found to enhance the nutritional intake of clients, to reduce food insecurity, and even to provide valuable social contact through the delivery person's brief visit.[24]

CONTINUING CARE RETIREMENT COMMUNITIES

For seniors who remain healthy, independent living facilities and self-created retirement communities can be an effective low-cost approach to fostering social engagement, intellectual activity, and a sense of usefulness and purpose. However, a different, more structured model, the continuing care retirement community (CCRC), merits serious consideration because it offers more services and a guaranteed availability of higher levels of care as one's medical needs change. A central feature of CCRCs is that they have independent living, assisted living, and nursing home care all in the same campus. CCRCs are not an option for low-income individuals because of their high entry and monthly fees. However, those with strong savings or considerable home equity should give CCRCs serious thought.

My Own CCRC Visits

While investigating options for my elderly father and researching this book, I visited several CCRCs. The first CCRC was in an urban setting with premier medical centers, a large university, and several cultural institutions nearby. It consisted of one multifloor building that offered 100 independent living apartments and 30 assisted living units. Those needing temporary or permanent nursing care were referred to an affiliated facility a mile away.

A tour of the CCRC revealed wood paneling, luxurious carpeting, two attractive dining rooms, several beautifully appointed common rooms, a roof-top terrace with a garden, an exercise room, a library, and an art studio. The independent living suites were spacious and airy with ample light and storage space, and many were newly renovated.

I had done extensive reading prior to my visits, so I was prepared for the very high initial entry fees and monthly charges that all of the facilities required. At this CCRC, entry fees that are 75 percent refundable upon leaving the CCRC or upon death, ranged from $170,000 to $402,000, depending on the size and features of the apartment. As an alternative, residents could opt for lower entry fees that ranged from $75,000 to $347,000 that were spread over 72 months. The lower entry fees were partially refundable only if the resident left or died before the end of 72 months. For example, if a resident died after 60 months, her estate would receive an amount representing payments for the last 12 months of the 72-month period, that is, one-sixth of the entry fee. In addition to paying an entry fee, CCRC residents pay monthly fees. At this CCRC, the lowest was $1,872 per month for an efficiency apartment, and the highest was $3,876 for a two-bedroom unit. If a second person shares the living quarters, both the entry fee and monthly fee are higher. Fees for assisted living and nursing care were even higher by considerable amounts.

A second CCRC was situated in a rural setting, featuring a beautiful campus of over 100 acres that was home to just over 300 residents. There were ponds, walking trails, an abundance of green space, and many gardens cultivated by residents. Independent housing was available in cottages or apartment buildings, and all activities and meetings took place in a large, central building so that community members would come together as often as possible. The building included a library, woodworking shop, several restaurants, a game room, a large swimming pool and fitness center, and a medical clinic, all of which were being used by many residents during my visit. The same building also included 48 attractive assisted living units and 48 nursing care rooms so that residents in these wings continued to be part of the community and could easily access activities. A child daycare center on premises allowed elderly residents to help care for young children and contributed to the lively environment.

At this CCRC, the entry fee for a "platinum plan" that covered all levels of care a resident might need at no extra charge ranged from $92,000 to $423,500 for single occupancy, and singles' monthly fees ranged from $2,514 to $4,702. For double occupancy, platinum plan entry fees ranged from $210,500 to $472,000, and monthly fees ranged from $4,404 to $6,230. Less comprehensive plans that would require additional payments for assisted living or nursing care could be obtained at reduced costs, with entry fees starting at $32,000 and monthly fees as low as $1,408 for a studio apartment. Plans with partially refundable entry fees were somewhat more expensive.

I also visited two CCRCs in suburban settings, both of which had large, beautifully landscaped campuses. They offered independent living residents the option of either villas or apartments that were adjacent to the community building. One was a high-end CCRC, with an emphasis on luxury. Its entry fees for singles were 75 percent refundable, beginning at $251,000 and reaching as high as $603,000, and its monthly fees ranged from $2,707 to $4,763. Monthly fees rose if the resident moved to assisted living. The second suburban CCRC was more modest in terms of décor, architecture, and apartment size but also had the most reasonable fees. The singles' entry fees for a life care plan were $73,000 to $313,000 and monthly fees were $1,767 to $3,116. With a life care plan, a resident would not need to pay additional fees if he or she moved to the assisted living or nursing home wings of the CCRC.

The CCRCs had much in common. Their fees generally include weekly housekeeping service, most utilities, scheduled transportation, maintenance, a 24-hour emergency call system, 24-hour security, all activities, and a dining allowance. The meals covered by the fees ranged from whatever you could buy for $200 a month to one meal of your choice every day. Applicants for residency undergo a financial screening, but all CCRC officials assured me that if residents exhaust their money despite being responsible about their finances, they are allowed to stay, and their expenses are covered by a charitable foundation or fund.

The administrators with whom I spoke emphasized that the staff knows residents well and everyone contributes to ensuring the members' well-being. The CCRCs I visited had large staffs, and several mentioned that they employed 200 to 300 people, though many of them worked part time. Because residents interact regularly with security officers, housekeepers, dining employees, and the CCRC's social workers and health care staff, any difficulty or decline is likely to be quickly detected. Those needing extra assistance while remaining in independent living may turn to an in-home care agency that is affiliated with the CCRC and hire an aide for $15 to $20 an hour.

Each CCRC had dementia patients among its nursing care residents. In several cases, these individuals were fully integrated into the community and wore a bracelet or anklet that tracked their movements for their own safety. In other cases, they lived in a unit with locked doors so they could not wander away from the building.

Upon visiting the CCRCs, I was handed several weekly newsletters with lengthy daily activity lists. These included scheduled transportation to medical and shopping destinations, arts and crafts, exercise classes, games, movies, concerts, coffee and ice cream socials, and lectures. The facilities that were closest to institutions of higher learning benefited from their cultural offerings, and residents could attend university events or even audit classes.

All of the CCRCs allowed residents to enjoy significant self-governance, with residents' councils and numerous committees.

In each case, I left with at least one concern. In two of the CCRCs, the many common rooms, hallways, and lobbies were generally empty. This observation caused me to wonder about whether the CCRC in fact created a robust social environment for its residents. By contrast, the community building in the other two CCRCs was bustling with activity, and I saw people chatting and smiling wherever I went.

The low point of a tour at one facility was the assisted living floor, which was shabby and had not been renovated in decades. My tour guide showed me the door to the "spa" room in which residents are bathed, but upon questioning, admitted that assistance with baths was offered only twice a week for those who could not wash themselves. At another CCRC, I was told that the aide-to-patient ratio in the skilled nursing wing was nine or 10 to one and that the nurses were responsible for 25 patients each, which seemed like an overwhelming patient load.

At the rural CCRC, those wishing to access the world-class medical facilities in the closest large city had to make special transportation arrangements for which they paid separately, and they had to travel approximately 35 miles. In addition, when I asked about religious services at this facility, I was told that they were available for several religious groups. However, because only 15 of the 300 residents were Jewish, no Jewish services were held, and the closest synagogue was 30 minutes away. This would have clearly been a drawback for my father, a retired rabbi. The answer to this casual question emphasized to me how important it is to research all aspects of the community and to spend as much time as possible at CCRCs of interest.

CCRC Benefits

There are approximately 2,000 CCRCs in the United States, serving close to 600,000 residents.[25] High-quality CCRCs can constitute an excellent living alternative for seniors. CCRCs feature a continuum of care, ranging from independent living to assisted living to skilled nursing homes, generally all in the same campus. Residents who move into a CCRC live in apartments, cottages, townhouses, or single-family homes, depending on the choices available at the facility. Ideally, CCRCs offer a large variety of services. These can include meals; social, educational, and other recreational programs; scheduled transportation; exercise facilities and classes; resident health clinics with nursing, physician, pharmacy, and physical and occupational therapy services; beauty salons; religious services; libraries; restaurants; guest accommodations; and more.[26] Thus, residents do not have to leave campus for the purposes of daily living. Moreover, scheduled transportation enables even those who do not drive to visit destinations such as nearby theaters, museums, shopping centers, medical specialists, and places of worship.

CCRCs often work hard to enable seniors to remain physically active and intellectually engaged and to retain a sense of meaning and purpose in their lives. Some are located near beaches or golf courses, and many are affiliated with religious groups or other social and community organizations. A particularly creative trend is the establishment of CCRCs on or near university campuses. Approximately 50 such communities existed as of 2010, and 50 more were planned. This arrangement enables seniors to take classes, attend cultural and sporting events, volunteer, and mentor students.[27]

A good CCRC can provide an ideal solution for seniors, especially those without family members who can frequently visit and care for them. Life can be active, rich, and fulfilling. In the words of one satisfied resident, "It's like being on a cruise. . . . You don't have to change the sheets, and there's always something to do."[28] A ready social circle is available, and in times of need, care and support can be provided by close friends in the community and professional staff members, including care coordinators.

A study of CCRCs and social integration concluded that moving to a CCRC enhanced "both objective connectedness and perceptions of being integrated." The researchers, who interviewed 92 residents at a CCRC in upstate New York in 1997 enthusiastically described their findings as follows:

> New residents both visit more with neighbors and volunteer more than they did prior to their relocation. They also feel more integrated, especially those most at risk of isolation (residents who are older, in poor health, or single females). . . . [A CCRC] offers availability and accessibility to important ways to remain connected as one ages.[29]

Another study of CCRC residents concluded that "health-related quality of life and engagement in discretionary activities is positively related among CCRC residents."[30] Thus, CCRC residents who are engaged in a rich array of activities are likely to enjoy better physical and psychological health than their contemporaries who do not have similar opportunities.

In theory at least, anxiety about the future is alleviated by the knowledge that the CCRC is home for life, even if one has to move among different components of the campus because of deteriorating health.[31] Thus, seniors can avoid social isolation and maintain many of their friendships and support networks as they seek higher levels of care.[32] CCRCs may also spare couples the trauma of separation if one spouse's health deteriorates to the point of needing nursing home care, since that facility will be within easy reach of the other spouse's residence. Some CCRCs have special wings dedicated to dementia and Alzheimer's patients and offer state-of-the-art memory care.

Close friends and dedicated staff members can encourage and support residents in making appropriate decisions about difficult matters such as giving up driving or seeking higher levels of care. By contrast, seniors who live independently without strong support networks may unwisely delay such steps and suffer adverse or even catastrophic consequences as a result. Furthermore, residents who need home care, assisted living, or nursing home services at the CCRC can be frequently visited by on-campus friends, who can serve the role of quality-of-care overseers and advocates.

 CCRC residents should enjoy opportunities for self-governance, should feel empowered to voice grievances without fear of retaliation, and should have problems redressed by a responsive management. In one reported case, for example, a CCRC reversed an unpopular policy that restricted some of its eateries to independent living residents and excluded those in assisted living and nursing home care. This policy, which was purportedly motivated by concerns about risks to frail patients and institutional liability, at times prevented close friends and even spouses from eating their meals together. In light of protests, the facility altered its policy to allow anyone to enjoy the eateries after signing a liability waiver, obtaining a doctor's permission, and undergoing a basic health screening.[33]

The average age of new residents in CCRCs is 80.[34] This is likely because living in a CCRC is relatively expensive, and many people worry that their savings will run out if they spend too many years there. Among the four CCRCs that I visited, new residents were slightly younger. An administrator at one told me that the average age at entry was 76 at her facility. Others were less specific and stated that the average move-in range was mid- to late seventies.

Moving to a high-quality CCRC can be the most comprehensive solution to the challenges of living well in old age. A national survey of 3,647 family members of CCRC residents revealed that 77 percent of them were "likely" or "very likely" to consider moving to a CCRC in the future.[35] Their interest in CCRCs was strongly influenced by their family members' positive experiences. Nevertheless, a move to a CCRC will be daunting or entirely impossible for many people because of its high cost.

CCRC Costs and Financial Risk

Residents are required to pay entrance fees generally ranging from $80,000 to $750,000 or even $1 million, with an average of $250,000, according to some estimates.[36] Entrance fees depend in part on the size and type of living unit selected and the contract format.

Typically, the entrance fee is refundable in whole or in part if residents die or move out, but refunds may be granted only once the unit is occupied by someone else. CCRCs may establish policies of full refunds (minus a fixed charge), partial refunds, or declining scale refunds and may designate a period of time after which no money will be refunded.[37]

In addition, residents must pay monthly charges that can range from less than $1,500 to over $10,000 and are subject to change. CCRCs may also impose additional fees for the various services they provide.[38] Residents can expect modest annual increases in their monthly fees that allow for building upkeep and renovation. One CCRC administrator told me that any facility that does not review its fees regularly in order to adopt "cost of living" increases is suspect and likely is not well maintained. However, institutions that experience financial stress may raise their fees considerably or begin charging for amenities that were initially free, unless price modifications are prohibited in the CCRC contract. Seniors who are accustomed to living in a home that is paid off and to enjoying a relatively low cost of living may be particularly wary of incurring high monthly expenses.

Three or four different contract options are available for CCRCs. Some facilities offer only one option and others offer multiple alternatives.

- A life care or extensive contract (type A) is the high-end option that includes all housing, residential services, and amenities and allows residents to enjoy the benefits of assisted living, medical treatment, and skilled nursing care without additional costs. Under this model, residents are entitled to lifetime services at all necessary levels of care without incurring monthly fee increases because of changes in their health status. Residents choosing type A contracts will have the advantage of predictable costs but may pay large sums of money for services they end up not using.
- Modified contracts (type B) include housing, residential services, amenities, and specified sets of health care services (e.g., 30 or 60 days of assisted living or nursing care). Entrance and monthly fees are lower than under type A contracts, but additional money is charged for extra services once those that are included are exhausted.
- Fee-for-service (type C) contracts typically feature even lower entrance and monthly fees and include housing, residential services, and amenities but no health care services. Residents are guaranteed access to assisted living and skilled nursing but must pay for them at market rates.
- Rental agreements (type D) allow seniors to rent housing on a monthly or annual basis and live in the CCRC. All services are paid for on a fee-for-services basis, and access to assisted living or nursing care may not be guaranteed. Type D contracts may require no entrance fees, and lower monthly charges cover housing only.[39]

In some cases, CCRCs offer equity agreements that enable individuals to own their CCRC house, condominium, or townhome. Residents or their heirs can then sell the property to age- and income-appropriate buyers.[40]

In many cases, a portion of the entrance fee and monthly fees can be recognized as a prepaid health care expense and thus is tax-deductible as a medical cost.* One CCRC that I visited provided a sheet that specified that the 2012 deduction for that facility was 20.7 percent. Residents should consult tax or financial advisers concerning this potential deduction.

The financial and organizational structure of CCRCs varies. The majority are nonprofit, but an increasing number are operated by for-profit entities. CCRCs may have endowment funds and extensive donor development programs.[41] Some are independent and are limited to one site. Others are owned by a parent company that operates multiple CCRCs. Multisite organizations can benefit from economies of scale, have more opportunities to learn from experience, and can spread risk among the different facilities so that if one temporarily experiences financial difficulties, it can be subsidized by income from facilities that are thriving. However, their disadvantages include increased bureaucracy, nonlocalized decisions about individual CCRCs, and multiple facilities competing for limited resources.[42]

Those considering CCRCs must understand that their investment is not without risk. During economic downturns, CCRCs' financial viability may be threatened by low occupancy rates in independent living units, which are the facilities' cash cows. For example, in 2011, CCRCs had a vacancy rate of 11 percent compared to a 6 percent vacancy rate in 2005,[43] though this discrepancy may be partially explained by the existence of fewer CCRCs in 2005. Although closures are rare, several filed for bankruptcy during the recession at the end of the 2000s.[44]

As an increasing number of baby boomers seek out CCRCs, they may become somewhat more affordable due to economies of scale and high occupancy rates. Entrance fees can often be covered by selling your home, but high monthly fees will likely remain a challenge for many.

According to some sources, CCRCs work hard to ensure that residents are not forced to leave in the face of depleted financial resources. Instead, management may apply the refundable portion of the entrance fee toward monthly payments or may provide opportunities for other residents to make voluntary contributions that support those in need. Some are able to offer other forms of financial aid thanks to ambitious fund-raising activities.[45]

So, are CCRCs unaffordable for people who are not wealthy? Not necessarily. Many seniors should be able to cover entry fees with proceeds from the sale of their homes. Furthermore, because monthly fees include a comprehensive set of services, CCRCs may minimize other living expenses. To illustrate, a single person's $3,000 fee for a one-bedroom apartment will include

---

*The amount depends on the CCRC's aggregate medical expenditures compared to its overall expenditures or overall income from resident fees.

numerous activities, transportation, many meals, utilities, an emergency call system, and more. Thus, if you do not seek to travel extensively or engage in other expensive leisure activities, ordinarily you may not need to spend much beyond the $3,000 fee each month.

During my own CCRC visits, I asked administrators to estimate the net worth of individuals who are good candidates for a CCRC, but they declined to provide any numbers. One, however, told me that a very rough rule of thumb is that residents' assets should be worth at least twice the entry fee, and their monthly incomes (from social security, pension, investments, etc.) should equal at least twice the monthly fee in order to cover living expenses, such as medical care and travel.

Other Concerns

Seniors may find it very difficult to leave beloved homes and familiar surroundings in which they have lived for decades. Moving will be especially daunting if it means seeing dear friends and relatives much less frequently. At the same time, those who are eager to live in a CCRC may find that their CCRC of choice has a waiting list that takes up to two years to clear. Consequently, it is important to begin researching CCRCs well in advance of being ready to move to one and to be prepared to delay the transition.

Consumers should also be aware that CCRCs are often underregulated by government authorities. Although the nursing homes and assisted living facilities located within CCRCs are governed by federal and state laws,[46] CCRCs as entities in and of themselves are subject to inconsistent oversight. Thus, states could go much further in regulating CCRCs in order to minimize the financial risk to residents and maximize the likelihood of the facilities' economic success.

As of 2010, 12 states had no CCRC-specific regulations. Only 17 states required CCRCs to provide information that would enable officials to assess their financial health and long-term outlook.[47] A government report found that the states that did regulate CCRCs established a range of requirements. The laws of different states featured some or all of the following:

- Licensing requirements, with varying degrees of financial disclosures and feasibility study standards;
- Annual submission of audited financial statements;
- Review of CCRC resident contracts;
- A mandated "cooling off period" during which dissatisfied residents may cancel their contracts and receive a refund of their full entrance fee, from which only specified costs can be deducted (typically the period ranges from prior to occupancy to one year after occupancy);

- Protection of CCRC residents' financial interests through (1) requirements that fees and deposits be escrowed, (2) specified criteria for raising monthly fees, and (3) authority to place liens or grant preferred status to claims in order to provide residents with recourse in the event of the CCRC's bankruptcy;
- Disclosure requirements concerning CCRCs' past, present, and anticipated future financial circumstances;
- Disclosure obligations concerning nonfinancial matters such as what policies operate when residents experience financial difficulties or whether the CCRC can transfer residents involuntarily to assisted living or nursing home care;
- Regulatory provisions that allow and encourage CCRC residents to form groups or councils for purposes of communicating with management and representing the interests of the residents at large;
- Preapproval of CCRC marketing and advertising material.[48]

Only one organization, the Commission on Accreditation of Rehabilitation Facilities–Continuing Care Accreditation Commission (CARF-CCAC), enables CCRCs to become accredited, and no states require this accreditation. In November 2014, CARF listed only 245 facilities as accredited on its website.[49]

It is possible that the availability of assisted living and nursing homes on campus can ironically be a disadvantage for residents. Management may be tempted to pressure residents to move to a higher level of care facility as soon as their health deteriorates or may actually require them to do so as a matter of policy. This may be particularly true if the CCRC will profit financially from such a move because of higher charges. Although counseling concerning appropriate care can be a valuable service that professional experts at the CCRC provide, individuals' autonomy should be respected. So long as residents are mentally competent, they should be free to remain in independent living settings and will hopefully accept assistance from home care workers. Admittedly, residents without children or other close family members who can influence them may present significant challenges for CCRCs if their mental or physical capacities deteriorate and they refuse to move to a higher level of care. In some cases, guardianship proceedings will need to be initiated, whereby a court will appoint a guardian to take over decision making for the resident.

Finally, it is important to note that there is currently a dearth of research on the efficacy of the CCRC model for the elderly. Some commentators postulate that transitioning to new housing for a higher level of care on the same campus might be just as difficult as moving across town because it still requires leaving one's home.[50] On the other hand, it seems sensible to assume that the transition would be considerably eased by frequent visits from members of the community and by the ability to travel around campus to familiar places. However, the evidence gap should be filled by scientific studies concerning the strengths and weaknesses of the CCRC model.

CCRC Hybrids

A small number of CCRC-type communities offer many of the benefits without the entrance fee. Independent living apartments are rented (not owned) by residents, and assisted living and sometimes nursing care rooms are also available onsite. Although these communities require no entrance fees, they charge for many services separately or have fairly high apartment rental costs to cover amenities such as meals, transportation, and programs. One such community, Calaroga Terrace in Portland, Oregon, which I had the occasion to visit in July 2013, advertised rental fees of $1,794 to $2,425 for a one-bedroom apartment and $3,095 to $3,495 for two-plus-bedroom apartments with no entry fees.[51] In addition, these CCRC hybrids may not guarantee residents acceptance into the assisted living or nursing care components of the facility even when residents truly need these higher levels of care.[52] Thus, those needing more care may be forced to move off campus.

Another CCRC alternative that appeals to some seniors is an emerging program called "CCRC without Walls." This program, which is available through at least a dozen CCRCs, allows clients to remain in their off-campus homes while taking advantage of many CCRC services. These include personal attention from a care coordinator, in-home meals, transportation, health clubs, social events, therapy, and, when necessary, assisted living or nursing home care. Members pay entrance fees and monthly fees, but they are lower than those paid by full CCRC residents. According to the *New York Times*, entrance fees range from $20,000 to $70,000 and monthly fees are $250 to $800.[53] To maintain the financial viability of the program, CCRCs without Walls generally accept only individuals who are healthy, competent, and functioning independently so that they do not need immediate institutional or other intensive care. CCRCs without Walls may not fully combat the problem of social isolation if participants do not frequently go to the campus and become involved in activities. However, the programs may address many of the needs of aging individuals at a more reasonable cost than CCRC residency.

RETIREMENT COMMUNITY PREPAREDNESS CHECKLIST

- Middle-aged individuals who are well-off financially should consider future CCRC residency and keep its cost in mind as they make their financial spending and saving choices. If CCRCs are not appealing or are out of reach, as they will inevitably remain for many, other forms of retirement communities, such as independent living residences, 55-plus communities, NORCs, and village networks should be investigated. What is critical is to find an environment that will facilitate staying active physically, mentally, and socially for as long as possible.

- For seniors living independently or in informal retirement communities, explore nearby senior centers that can provide various forms of support, including socially and intellectually enriching activities.
- Keep the importance of having a robust social circle in mind. The transition to a retirement community can be eased by moving to a facility in the same city, moving with a group of friends, or selecting one in which friends are already living.
- If you are considering a retirement community for yourself or loved ones, ask about the existence of waiting lists, because the more popular and reputable retirement communities may require long waits. For example, during several CCRC visits, I was told that it could take up to 18 to 24 months to obtain a living unit after making an initial deposit.
- Finding an appropriate retirement community should involve significant research. Once you identify a facility of interest, you should spend significant time there to determine whether it is a good fit. CCRCs in particular often have guest suites that can be rented for a few nights, and an actual stay at the facility for at least two days is very helpful in the decision-making process. It is only by spending time at the retirement community and speaking with residents that you can get a real feel for the place.
- If you are considering a CCRC, be sure to visit its assisted living and nursing home components and to speak with residents about them. How do residents fare in these units? To what extent do they remain integrated into the community? Are these attractive settings? Do those who move to them from independent living feel stigmatized? Do people try to hide their frailties at all costs in order to avoid being transferred to assisted living or nursing care?
- If you are considering a CCRC, a report by the U.S. Senate Special Committee on Aging suggests that you investigate the following:
  - The CCRC's fee structure, including entrance fee refund policies;
  - Ownership structure: for-profit vs. nonprofit and stand-alone vs. one of several owned by a parent company;
  - The facility's financial performance;
  - Protection against involuntary transfer to different levels of care or to an off-campus location;
  - Opportunities for residents to participate in management decisions, to voice grievances, and to have their concerns addressed;
  - Circumstances in which contracts can be rescinded or canceled;

-     ○ CCRC accreditation.[54]
- Consult other resources that provide extensive information about CCRCs. These include the AARP's "What to Ask and Observe When Visiting Continuing Care Retirement Communities," CARF-CCAC's "Consumer Guide to Understanding Financial Performance and Reporting in Continuing Care Retirement Communities," and the California Advocates for Nursing Home Reform's "Points to Consider for CCRC Consumers."[55]
- Once you select a retirement community and have a contract in hand, read it carefully. You would also be well advised to consult a lawyer prior to signing it if it is complicated (as in the case of CCRCs) or you have questions about it. You should also consult a financial or tax adviser to determine whether any deductions are available and whether moving to the facility requires you to change any of your financial practices.

3

Help with Money, Care, and Home Management

During our phone conversations, my sister often told me how much time she spent paying my father's bills, filling his pill boxes, scheduling his medical appointments, accompanying him to doctors' offices, taking care of repairs, and much more. My sister's help enabled my father, who was in his late eighties, to continue residing in his house, with added assistance from paid caregivers. Although I felt somewhat guilty about the disproportionate burden she bore because she was the one who lived close to our father, I am grateful that he had her devoted assistance.

What about those of us who will not have loved ones available to offer daily or weekly support? Who might provide help with these critical matters? Thankfully, professional services are increasingly becoming available to meet seniors' needs.

DAILY MONEY MANAGERS

Daily money managers (DMM) offer a range of services to seniors. These most commonly include the following:

- Bill paying, including calls to payees regarding incorrect bills and preparation of checks for clients to sign.
- Balancing checkbooks and maintaining organization of bank records.

- Preparing and delivering bank deposits.
- Organizing tax documents and other paperwork.
- Negotiating with creditors.
- Deciphering medical insurance papers and verifying proper processing of claims.
- Providing referrals to legal, tax, and investment professionals.[1]

DMMs generally visit the homes of elderly clients in order to assist them with financial tasks. In addition to attending to the matters listed above, DMMs may do the following: help clients make Medicare enrollment decisions; review documents relating to estate planning, power of attorney, and beneficiaries; assist in identifying the best rates for cable, phone, and other services; and even transport clients to appointments.[2]

Daily money management is an emerging profession, and the American Association of Daily Money Managers (AADMM) had over 750 members as of 2014.[3] The AADMM website enables users to search for DMMs by geographic location. Fees range from $50 to $150 or more per hour.[4]

The DMM field, however, is not regulated by state or federal authorities. This is of concern because DMMs have access to clients' checkbooks, financial information, and other sensitive materials, and thus dishonest individuals would have ample opportunity to exploit the elderly. The AADMM publishes a code of ethics, but there is no enforcement mechanism that can ensure compliance.[5]

It is therefore very important to employ trustworthy individuals. Recommendations from people who are familiar with the DMM you are considering can be particularly valuable. DMM certification is another quality indicator and is available through the AADMM. Applicants for certification must have a high school diploma and 1,500 hours of DMM experience over the prior three years. They must also undergo a criminal background check and pass a test consisting of 100 multiple-choice questions concerning bill paying, bookkeeping, taxes, and other relevant matters.[6] As of late 2014, however, the list of certified DMMs published on the AADMM website was short, including only 79 professionals.[7]

Another safeguard is to ensure that the DMM is bonded and employed by an organization with an insurance policy that will provide appropriate compensation for theft, fraud, and other forms of malpractice.[8] Elderly people who use DMMs can also take the following precautions: limit the money available in the checking account that the DMM will use, sign all checks themselves, and review all financial statements or ask a trusted friend or relative to do so.[9] Automating as many payments as possible will also reduce the DMM's workload, decrease charges, and limit opportunities for errors or dishonesty.

GERIATRIC CARE MANAGERS

Geriatric care managers (GCMs) provide an array of services that can be invaluable for seniors who lack sufficient family support. GCMs are generally social workers, nurses, gerontologists, psychologists, or other human services professionals[10] who focus on assessment, monitoring, planning, problem solving, and advocacy for elderly clients and their caregivers.[11] More specifically, geriatric care management can be defined as "a service that assesses an individual's medical and social service needs, then coordinates assistance from paid service providers and unpaid help from family and friends to enable persons with disabilities to live with as much independence as possible."[12]

The first encounter with a GCM involves a comprehensive assessment, after which a variety of services can be provided. The National Association of Professional Geriatric Care Managers (NAPGCM) website asserts that GCMs may do all of the following:

- Assist in selecting appropriate housing or residential settings;
- Determine what home care services are necessary and assist in monitoring them;
- Attend doctor appointments with clients, facilitate communication with doctors, and monitor the client's compliance with medical instructions;
- Provide opportunities for clients to participate in social, recreational, or cultural events and activities;
- Provide referrals to elder law attorneys or consult with them;
- Provide expert testimony for purposes of court proceedings;
- Oversee bill paying and review financial affairs in consultation with accountants or the client's power of attorney;
- Help clients obtain federal and state entitlements and benefits;
- Assess the home environment and offer recommendations to enhance clients' safety and general welfare.[13]

According to the Institute for the Future of Aging Services, in 2002, one-third of seniors who retained GCMs used their services for four to nine years and another third had employed them for over 10 years.[14]

The NAPGCM had 2,037 members in 2013. Like the DMM specialty, geriatric care management is an emerging profession with considerable room for growth. All members are required to hold one of four certifications: care manager certified, certified case manager, certified advanced social work case manager, and certified social work case manager.[15]

The NAPGCM website enables users to search for local GCMs.[16] GCMs typically charge $75 to $250 per hour for their services.[17]

GCM use has been associated with a number of benefits for the elderly. These include fewer emergency department visits, hospitalizations, and falls;

increased ability to follow instructions concerning medications; and a greater probability of delaying or avoiding a move to assisted living or a nursing home.[18] GCMs may also help decrease depression in the elderly and relieve caregiver burdens and stress.[19]

ELDER LAW ATTORNEYS

Elder law attorneys can assist not only the elderly themselves but also those who are wise enough to want to plan ahead of time for old age. In the words of one lawyer, they can steer clients away from being "geriatric gamblers" and "planning procrastinators" to being "pragmatic planners."[20]

Elder law attorneys may provide both legal assistance and general care coordination for aging clients. The legal matters that an elder law attorney can address include the following:

- Health and personal care planning, including advance directives;
- Financial planning, housing matters, and tax issues (income, estate, and gift tax);
- Planning for a well spouse when the other requires long-term care, including asset protection and the attainment of public benefits such as Medicare or Medicaid and veterans' benefits;
- Obtaining a court-appointed guardian for a person who has lost decision-making ability;
- Avoiding the need for a guardian by naming a substitute decision maker in a power of attorney document so that the named individual can assume decision-making responsibility if the need arises;
- Defending residents' rights in residential facilities such as nursing homes;
- Handling employment and retirement concerns;
- Drafting and handling wills, trusts, estate planning, and probate;
- All other legal planning for aging, illness, and incapacity.[21]

Some entrepreneurial attorneys are adopting a "holistic approach" and including other elder care specialists among their staff. They thus create multidisciplinary practices by employing nurses, geriatric care managers, insurance specialists, social workers, investment advisers, and others who can provide a comprehensive package of services to older clients.[22]

The National Elder Law Foundation website allows users to search for certified elder law attorneys in their own state. The National Academy of Elder Law Attorneys had over 4,500 members in 2010,[23] and the organization provides resources and support for practitioners.[24] The American Bar Association has accredited the National Elder Law Foundation to certify lawyers as elder law attorneys. As of 2014, however, there were only 460 certified elder law attorneys in the United States.[25] Those certified must demonstrate that they have practiced law for the preceding five years and handled at least 60 elder law matters on which they spent a minimum of 16 hours per week on average during the past three years. They also must have at least 45 hours of continuing legal education in elder law during the preceding three years. Certification further involves a full-day examination and must be renewed every five years.[26]

Chapter 4 provides an extensive discussion of the legal documents you should have to be prepared for your later years or for loss of decision-making capacity at any point in your life.

ORGANIZING, ADAPTING, AND SELLING YOUR HOME

As my parents reached their mid-seventies, my sisters and I became increasingly concerned about their ability to stay in their large, two-story home. Occasionally, they seemed unsteady on their feet, and a few times, they fell. We worried about their ability to maneuver up or down the stairs and even to get in and out of the shower safely. Yet, they resisted moving to a smaller, one-story residence because it seemed like an overwhelming task. They had accumulated decades' worth of possessions and papers, and they lacked the energy to cull through them. It took us years to convince them to move, and then it took a long time to sell their house. It turns out that there were plenty of professionals who could have helped them organize their home, prepare it for sale, and adapt it to their needs while they waited to make their decision and purchase a condominium. If only we had known!

Adapting Your Home

People who wish to remain in their homes but have mobility or other impairments can modify their residences to better suit their needs. For example, you might make the following changes:

- Install grab bars for support in the shower, over the tub, and by the toilet;
- Buy a raised toilet seat;
- Widen doorways and passageways to accommodate a walker or wheelchair;
- Install a chair lift for the stairs;
- Install a ramp to avoid using steps to enter the house;
- Buy specialized furniture, such as adjustable beds and recliners.

Such changes can make the home significantly safer and reduce the likelihood of falls and trips to the emergency room. For advice about modifying your home, you can consult an occupational therapist. Websites such as Healthgrades.com and OccupationalTherapist.com allow users to search for local occupational therapists.

Personal Emergency Response and Detection Systems

A particularly useful addition to the home of a frail individual is a personal emergency response system. These devices allow elderly people to contact 911 or family members by pushing a button on a bracelet or pendant. If an emergency occurs in the house or immediately outside of it, such as a fall, the client need only push the button to send a signal to a console that automatically dials the emergency number. As of 2014, approximately 2 million individuals had such systems in the United States and generally paid for them out of pocket as an expense that is not covered by insurance.[27] Nevertheless, these devices can save clients money by reducing the need for coverage by in-home care aides because users know there will be a quick response when the need arises even if they are alone at home.

Unfortunately, some people who have personal emergency response and detection systems rarely wear them or do not activate them even when appropriate. Most commonly, they underutilize them because they don't believe they need them, don't want to admit that they are vulnerable, are worried about bothering family members, or wish to avoid hospital visits at all costs. Consequently, some vendors are developing technologies that do not require users to operate them in any way. These include in-home monitoring systems that do not need to be worn and pendants with fall-detection capabilities that operate automatically and do not need to be manually activated.

Seniors may worry that having a personal emergency response and detection system will reduce their social contact because family and friends will check on them less often. This may be a valid concern in some cases, but overall, the devices have been found to be effective when used, and users indicate they are highly satisfied with them. They enhance seniors' sense of security, allow them to remain independent longer, and even shorten hospital stays because patients receive immediate attention when they are injured.[28]

Professional Organizers

Professional organizers will help you organize just about anything. Some focus on assisting businesses and others on helping people with their homes. Some even specialize in serving particular populations, such as seniors.

Organizing can be useful at any time, especially prior to moving out of the home. A professional could help you or your loved one downsize and discard possessions and paperwork that have been accumulated over decades.

Homeowners, who do this work with or without professional assistance can save their survivors a lot of stress and agony later on.

According to the National Association of Professional Organizers' website (yes, they have their own national association):

> An organizer's services can range from designing an efficient closet to organizing a cross-country move. For homeowners, he or she might offer room-by-room space planning and reorganization, estate organization, improved management of paperwork and computer files, systems for managing personal finances and other records, and/or coaching in time-management and goal-setting.[29]

The association has approximately 4,000 members and offers an annual conference, a blog, and educational teleclasses. Its website features a directory that makes it easy for users to locate nearby professional organizers. A quick search reveals that many organizers have a knack for clever names. For example, who could resist employing a service named "Leff's Last Re-Sort" or "Can the Clutter"?[30]

Home Staging

Once you are ready to sell your home or the home of an elderly loved one, you might want to consult a home stager, especially if the residence has not been recently updated. Home stagers assist customers by "accentuating positive architectural features, opening up spaces, neutralizing colors, and conveying comfort . . . [to] present your property in its best light."[31]

As my parents learned after initially having difficulty selling their house, stripping off old wallpaper, applying fresh, light-colored paint, and replacing dark appliances with white ones can make a big difference. The International Association of Home Staging Professionals has a search icon on its website that enables users to locate stagers in their area. If you do not want to use a stager or cannot afford one, you can ask your real estate agent for suggestions as to how to make the home more appealing to buyers and hope that he or she has a good eye. Cosmetic changes may both make the home sell more quickly and help you get a higher price for it.

EMPLOYING ELDER CARE SERVICE PROFESSIONALS

The benefits of employing reliable daily money managers (DMMs), geriatric care managers (GCMs), elder law attorneys, and experts who can assist elderly people manage at home can be considerable. These professionals can help seniors maintain their independence and avoid having to move to assisted living or nursing facilities. One 2012 study estimated that seniors who lived at home until death with the help of DMMs and GCMs saved an average of $60,000 in total costs by avoiding nursing homes.[32] The lifetime cost of care management averaged $108,810, and that of DMM services was $8,656. DMMs and GCMs may save clients further costs by paying clients' bills so they avoid costly errors, late fees, and interest; assisting them with applying for government benefits; and identifying free or inexpensive community resources for clients.

In addition, DMMs can potentially combat elder financial abuse. Women over 80 who have lost their life partners, are lonely, and suffer from deteriorating health are particularly vulnerable.[33] Elders may be deceived by strangers who call them or knock on their doors, tenants who stop paying rent, caregivers who demand loans or gifts, and even family members who take advantage of a relative's frailty. Seniors who use computers but are naive about spam and fraudulent financial schemes may be victimized by electronic means. Skilled professionals who oversee elderly individuals' financial affairs should be able to save their clients from being duped by exploiters.[34]

Those without children or other dedicated, unpaid helpers need not be left to manage their affairs completely on their own or fail to manage them at all. DMMs, GCMs, organizers, and occupational specialists can provide much-needed assistance to elderly individuals with physical ailments that limit their functionality, such as arthritis or deteriorating vision, and to those who simply no longer wish to take care of certain mundane tasks. Unfortunately, however, elderly people whose cognitive abilities decline will likely be unable to hire, work with, and supervise professionals on their own.

When the client is mentally impaired, the success of professionals' services generally depends on the availability of children or others who can explain the client's needs, offer access to documents and accounts, and provide some degree of oversight. For the childless, this role could be fulfilled by trusted friends or more distant relatives. Paid professionals can relieve much of the burden that would otherwise be borne by unpaid caregivers so that the latter need not attend to the elderly person's affairs on a day-to-day basis. Planned retirement communities, as discussed in Chapter 2, or elder law attorneys may have DMMs and GCMs on staff or be able to provide reliable referrals.

For individuals who live alone without a close-knit social circle, the challenge will be to recognize that their mental capacity is declining and that they need the aid of human services professionals. Consequently, it is all the more important for the elderly to maintain social bonds and frequent contact with trusted friends or relatives. Living in a retirement community or otherwise in close proximity to loved ones can be critical to seniors' welfare. In addition, seniors would be wise to form a relationship with an elder law attorney and/ or a GCM while their full faculties are intact so that a skilled expert will know them well, monitor them, and suggest interventions when appropriate.

In fact, consulting an elder law attorney would be a responsible step for every working person to take long before retirement. As discussed in Chapter 4, every individual should have a detailed will, living will, durable power of attorney for health care, and durable power of attorney for property and finances. Of particular relevance here, properly designated agents can coordinate the work of DMMs and GCMs for incapacitated persons.

As baby boomers age, we are likely to see growth in the emerging professions of DMMs, GCMs, and elder law attorneys. At the same time, let us hope that professional organizations and state governments will implement uniform and stringent certification and oversight requirements. DMMs and GCMs in particular have seniors' financial, physical, and emotional health in their hands. Clients should not have to gamble when hiring them and be left to guess about their quality and integrity.

HELP WITH MONEY, CARE, AND HOME MANAGEMENT PREPAREDNESS CHECKLIST

- If you or a loved one has trouble managing fiscal matters, consider hiring a daily money manager.
- Seniors without strong family support systems should consider hiring geriatric care managers.
- Consult an elder law attorney to ensure that you are legally prepared for your later years, as discussed more fully in Chapter 4.
- If you or a loved one is having trouble adapting, organizing, or selling a home, consider hiring professionals who can assist with these tasks: occupational therapists, organizers, and home stagers.
- When hiring professionals, opt for those who are members of their professional organizations, have undertaken relevant educational programs, and, if possible, are certified in their specialty.
- Have a personal emergency response and detection system installed in the home to ensure that you or your loved one can get immediate assistance in an emergency.

4

Essential Legal Planning

In Chapter 1, I discussed the woefully inadequate retirement savings that many Americans accrue during their working lives. Are we any better at legal preparedness for old age? Perhaps not surprisingly, the answer is no.

I remember a phone call I received from a friend who was in her seventies and was suffering a recurrence of an aggressive cancer. "I'm thinking I should have a will," she said and asked me to recommend a lawyer. I was shocked that this highly educated woman had not previously executed a will, especially given her age and medical history, but she is not alone. An alarming number of Americans do not have wills. According to 2013 statistics, only 43 percent of adults in their forties have prepared wills, and among individuals 70 and older, only 78 percent have wills.[1]

Thorough planning must include contemplation of worst-case scenarios, such as a temporary or permanent loss of mental faculties. Because almost 14 percent of individuals 70 and older suffer from dementia[2] and many others experience temporary incapacity resulting from illness or surgery, it is prudent to consider this possibility and formulate contingency plans. It is also wise to ensure that your assets will be distributed in accordance with your wishes after you die. Legal documents can serve all of these purposes.

ADVANCE DIRECTIVES FOR HEALTH CARE

I am a member of the ethics committee of University Hospitals in Cleveland, Ohio. In one meeting in 2013, we learned of a case in which a man came to the hospital with his daughter in order to undergo surgery to remove kidney stones. The anesthesiologist who spoke with the patient determined, based on the conversation, that the man had dementia and was not capable of providing informed consent to the procedure. The daughter volunteered to consent in place of her father but admitted that her father had not executed an advance directive naming her as his agent and that she had not been designated as her father's guardian by an Ohio court. Consequently, the patient was denied the surgery and sent home. The daughter was told that because her father's dementia would prevent him from executing a valid advance directive, he could not have this nonemergency operation until she obtained guardianship and thus legal authority to consent to his care. Appointment of a guardian, however, involves court proceedings and can take several months, during which the man's treatment would be delayed, and he could potentially suffer excruciating pain.[3] Although most states have default surrogates statutes that would allow close relatives to make medical decisions, Ohio's applies only to withdrawal or withholding of life-sustaining treatment.[4]

This unfortunate outcome could have been avoided if the patient had an advance directive, a document that allowed him to provide legally valid instructions concerning his health care if he became incapacitated.[5] Incapacity is generally defined as an inability to make and communicate informed decisions,[6] and determinations of incapacity are typically made by attending physicians.[7] An advance directive may include one or more of the following components: a living will, a durable power of attorney for health care, and an organ donation form, each of which will be discussed separately below.

Adults with decision-making capacity have the ability to consent to medical treatment and a right to refuse health care interventions, even if doing so will shorten their lives. On the other hand, patients who are mentally incapacitated, by definition, cannot make medical decisions. Researchers have found that over a quarter of elderly patients lose the ability to engage in decision making prior to death.[8] Before losing capacity, individuals may have strong views about the care they wish to receive in particular circumstances, and the prospect of having those wishes ignored can be heartbreaking. All individuals who seek to ensure that their preferences will be given deference even if they can no longer articulate them should prepare advance directives. As the example above illustrates, another reason to execute an advance directive is that in some circumstances, it may be difficult, if not impossible, for an incapacitated individual to obtain nonemergency care at all without this document.

All fifty states and the District of Columbia recognize advance directives, although the state laws differ in their particulars.[9] For example, the states vary as to their instructions for completing an advance directive, in some cases requiring notarization and in others asking for the signature of one or two witnesses.[10]

The Patient Self-Determination Act (PSDA) of 1990 establishes that all hospitals, long-term care facilities, home health agencies, hospice programs, and health maintenance organizations (HMOs) that receive Medicare and Medicaid payments must recognize patient advance directives. They must also:

- Ask patients at the time of admission if they have advance directives;
- Give patients written information about advance directives;
- Document patients' advance directives in their medical records;
- Comply with state law requirements concerning advance directives;
- Avoid discrimination against individuals based on their having or not having advance directives;
- Educate staff and the community about advance directives.[11]

Nevertheless, by now you probably will not be surprised to learn that relatively few Americans have taken advantage of this opportunity to plan for the future. Experts estimate that only 18 to 36 percent of adults have completed advance directives.[12]

This may be in part because the PSDA's requirements do not extend to individual physicians, and few physicians initiate discussions about advance directives. Physicians may feel pressed for time,* ill equipped to address the subject, or reluctant to raise a matter that patients might be loath to discuss.[13]

Middle-aged individuals should not wait for others to urge them to execute advance directives, but rather, should take the initiative themselves. Those who can afford to consult an attorney should do so, and lawyers will often include advance directives in an estate planning package for a very modest fee.[14] As an alternative, you may turn to web-based tools such as these popular sources:

Aging with Dignity's Five Wishes: http://www.agingwithdignity.org/forms/5wishes.pdf

CaringConnections:http://www.caringinfo.org/i4a/pages/index.cfm?pageid=3289. This source enables users to download state-specific advance directives.

---

*An early draft of the Patient Protection and Affordable Care Act, now popularly known as "Obamacare," included a provision titled "Advance Care Planning Consultation." The law would have enabled physicians to be paid for voluntarily advising Medicare patients about living wills, advance directives, and end-of-life care options. Unfortunately, this provision was abandoned in the face of baseless charges by Sarah Palin and others that it would lead to the establishment of "death panels" with authority to deprive the elderly and disabled of needed medical treatment. H.R. 3200, 11th Cong., 1st Sess. §1233 (2009).

Individuals can provide detailed instructions in their advance directives concerning their care preferences upon incapacity. In doing so, they may indicate that they wish to receive aggressive medical intervention for as long as possible or that, under certain circumstances, they want to decline any care beyond comfort measures. Most commonly, people use advance directives to request that their care be limited rather than instructing that everything always be done to prolong their lives regardless of their degree of incapacity.[15] The mechanisms for directing future medical care through legal documentation are discussed in detail below.

Living Wills

One important component of the advanced directive is the living will. Living wills allow individuals to specify the kinds of treatment they would wish to have in a limited set of circumstances: if they become terminally ill or permanently unconscious or are in a vegetative state.[16] Terminal illnesses are typically defined to include irreversible or incurable diseases or injuries leading to death. Some states elaborate and provide that there must be an absence of a reasonable probability of recovery or that death is anticipated within a short time after life-sustaining medical treatment is withheld.[17]

Because I live in Ohio, I will use its Living Will Declaration as an example. It enables individuals to state the following:

If I am in a terminal condition and unable to make my own health care decisions, I direct that my physician shall:
1. Administer no life-sustaining treatment, including CPR and artificially or technologically supplied nutrition or hydration; and
2. Withdraw such treatment, including CPR, if such treatment has started; and
3. Issue a DNR Order; and
4. Permit me to die naturally and take no action to postpone my death, providing me with only that care necessary to make me comfortable and to relieve my pain.

Similar choices can be made with respect to treatment if one is in a permanently unconscious state (rather than "in a terminal condition"), with more detailed instructions concerning artificial nutrition and hydration.[18]

Notably, the standard form in Ohio and many other states includes only instructions for withholding care. Some individuals will want their physicians to employ the opposite approach and do everything in order to prolong life, regardless of their medical condition. This choice, of course, is equally valid. However, individuals with this preference will need to work with an attorney in order to create a living will that is different from the standard form.

It is essential to realize that living wills apply only in limited circumstances, as described above. Consequently, they do not provide individuals with an opportunity for wide-ranging input into their care should they become incapacitated. Thus, it is important to have both a living will and a health care power of attorney, which, under some state laws, can be included in the same advance directive document.

Durable Power of Attorney for Health Care

A durable power of attorney for health care names an agent (also called a proxy) who will serve as the decision maker for an individual (the principal) anytime the principal is unable to make decisions for him- or herself, not just at the end of life. It is also useful to name one or more alternative agents who will assume responsibility if the original proxy becomes unavailable.

The Ohio Health Care Power of Attorney document lists a large number of decisions that are within the power of the agent but allows those signing the document to cross items off the list or to provide additional details concerning their wishes. For example, you can indicate that you want your agent to have authority to do the following:

- To consent to the administration of pain-relieving drugs, treatments, or procedures, including surgery, that aim to alleviate discomfort, even if they might hasten your death.
- To consent or refuse to consent to life-sustaining treatment, including nutrition and hydration if you are terminally ill.
- To consent or refuse to consent to any medical treatment.
- To request and review medical information regarding your mental or physical health.
- To consent to the disclosure of your medical information to other people, such as family members.
- To select, hire, and fire health care providers and service providers such as in-home care aides.
- To have you admitted or discharged from medical institutions such as a hospital, nursing home, assisted living facility, or hospice.

As is typical in many states,[19] Ohio limits the authority of the agent in several ways, and these limitations cannot be overridden:

- Your agent cannot order the withdrawal of life-sustaining treatment if you are not in a terminal condition or a permanently unconscious state. In addition, your agent can only instruct that life-sustaining treatment be withdrawn if two physicians have confirmed the diagnosis and have determined that you have no reasonable possibility of regaining the ability to make decisions.

- Your agent cannot order the withdrawal of any treatment that is given to you in order to make you more comfortable or to relieve pain.
- If you are pregnant, your agent cannot refuse treatment if doing so would end your pregnancy, unless the pregnancy or treatment would substantially endanger your life or two physicians determine that the fetus would not be born alive.
- Your agent cannot order the withdrawal of artificially supplied nutrition or hydration unless you are terminally ill or permanently unconscious and two physicians agree that nutrition or hydration will not provide comfort or relieve pain. In addition, you must specify in the document that you want nutrition and hydration to be withdrawn if you are permanently unconscious.
- Your agent cannot withdraw any treatment to which you previously consented unless your condition has significantly changed so that the treatment is far less beneficial to you or has failed to achieve its purpose.[20]

Advance directives can provide very detailed instructions for the health care proxy. A sample published in the *American Journal of Bioethics* addresses a variety of serious conditions separately and lists treatments that the principal may or may not want to receive. For example, one section addresses "moderate/severe dementia" that renders the person unable to care for him- or herself or to "remember things clearly." You can check boxes as to whether you would want to have kidney dialysis, mechanical ventilation, or a feeding tube for various lengths of time as well as cardiopulmonary resuscitation, medicines, surgery, and blood transfusions.[21]

The American Bar Association Commission on Law and Aging offers guidance as to how to choose a health care agent. The proxy should be a trustworthy individual who knows the principal well, fully understands his or her wishes after open discussions about care preferences, and can be a competent advocate even when faced with unresponsive health care providers or family members who have conflicting opinions about treatment plans. Furthermore, the agent must be able to follow the principal's wishes even if these wishes are contrary to his or her own beliefs. The proxy should be easily reachable and available when needed and willing to serve in this capacity for many years to come.[22]

Some individuals are ineligible to serve as proxies. Most commonly, states exclude (1) anyone younger than 18; (2) the principal's health care providers and their employees; and (3) the owners or operators of any health, residential, or community care facility that serves the principal, though spouses and close relatives can always be designated as agents.[23]

If you have different agents for health care and financial decisions, you should ensure that the two know each other, can communicate with each other, and fully understand your wishes. The health care proxy will need the cooperation of the financial proxy in order to pay for whatever care is selected. Family members should also be informed as soon as agents have been appointed in order to reduce the likelihood that they will later try to assert themselves as decision makers and create friction or conflict.[24]

Anatomical Gift Form

According to the U.S. Department of Health and Human Services, as of the end of October 2014, 124,113 people were waiting for an organ. During the first seven months of 2014, 16,884 transplants were performed, but because of persistent organ shortages, 21 people die each day while waiting for organs. One donor can save as many as eight lives because you can donate your kidneys, pancreas, liver, lungs, heart, intestines, bones, skin, heart valves, veins, and corneas.[25]

Many people believe that making anatomical gifts will render their lives (and deaths) more meaningful, but organ donation does not occur automatically. The best way to ensure consideration as an organ donor is to sign onto a state organ and tissue donor registry. These registries can be accessed through the government's organ donor website.* Many states' advance directive forms also enable individuals to indicate their desire to provide anatomical gifts upon death.[26] This part of the form may need to be sent to a particular agency, such as the state Department of Motor Vehicles, to ensure enrollment as a donor.[27] Not everyone who signs up ends up being a donor because your organs must be healthy enough to be donated and you must be a match for someone who needs an organ at the time of your death. However, without an anatomical gift form, your wishes may not be known and followed.

Some people have religious or other reasons for not becoming organ donors. However, many people have no objection to being organ donors or even affirmatively want to do so, but they do not take the trouble to fill out the form. This inaction costs lives. If you want to donate your organs after death (I promise, you won't need them anymore), please take a few minutes to do the paperwork. If you are creating other legal documents to prepare for possible incapacity and death, this is the perfect time to consider also filling out an organ donation form.

Advance Directive for Mental Health Treatment

Individuals with a history of mental illness may choose to prepare an advance directive that is specific to mental health treatment. People with capacity can

---

*Available at http://www.organdonor.gov/becomingdonor/stateregistries.html.

designate agents who will make mental health care decisions for them if they lose capacity permanently or temporarily and çan provide specific instructions concerning therapies that they wish or do not wish to receive. You can select one agent for mental health care and another for all other care, and if the agents are different, separate directives should be executed.[28] According to the National Resource Center on Psychiatric Advance Directives,[29] 25 states have enacted psychiatric advance directive statutes.*

An advance directive for mental health treatment should address matters such as:

- Which medications are acceptable and unacceptable to the patient;
- Facilities at which treatment can be provided;
- Which types of treatment the patient is willing to undergo (e.g., electroconvulsive treatment);
- Instructions concerning the temporary care of children or loved ones during the principal's incapacity.

Mental health advance directives may be especially useful because they are tailored to a particular condition or conditions with which you have experience. The course of treatment is predictable and you can be specific in your instructions.[30]

Nevertheless, only a small fraction of patients with mental illness have a psychiatric advance directive. This may be because most people are unaware of this advance directive option, and few educational initiatives focus on this matter.[31]

Patients should know, however, that many state statutes allow physicians to override treatment requests with which they disagree in some circumstances.[32] For example, Ohio's statute governing declarations for mental health treatment permits an override if the patient is committed and a court "orders treatment in a manner contrary to the declaration" or if an "emergency situation endangers the life or health of the declarant or others."[33]

BARRIERS TO ADVANCE DIRECTIVE IMPLEMENTATION

Unfortunately, the mere execution of an advance directive does not guarantee that one's wishes will be honored in the event of incapacity. Several

---

*As of 2013, the states included Arizona, Hawaii, Idaho, Illinois, Indiana, Kentucky, Louisiana, Maine, Maryland, Michigan, Minnesota, Montana, New Jersey, New Mexico, North Carolina, Ohio, Oklahoma, Oregon, Pennsylvania, South Dakota, Tennessee, Texas, Utah, Washington, and Wyoming.

barriers may prevent advance directives from being followed by health care providers.

Portability

Individuals may complete an advance directive in one state and then move to another state and forget to prepare a new directive. Whether or not their advance directives will be recognized by their new state will depend on state law. Many states provide for recognition of out-of-state directives, but others are silent on the matter.[34]

In addition, patients may give their advance directive to one physician or hospital but be treated at multiple facilities by numerous doctors, as often occurs late in life. If the patient becomes incapacitated but the physicians or institutions providing care at the time do not have a copy of the advance directive, the patient's proxy may not be contacted and his or her preferences may not be considered.[35]

Quality and Specificity of Instructions

According to one study, "directives often provide abstract guidance not easily translated to the nuanced contingencies of real-world patient care."[36] Many instructions are worded using medical terminology that patients do not fully understand and that causes severe problems for medical personnel. For example, laypeople may believe that the word "coma" means any nonresponse state, but in medicine it is characterized by precise criteria. Furthermore, some advance directives contain conditional instructions that depend on prognosis. The principal might be asked to select options that apply "if I am in a coma that would resolve within a year."[37] But prognosis is often impossible to predict with any degree of certainty, and doctors can provide no specific timetable for recovery.[38]

Yet another problem is that wishes are often expressed in absolute terms, such as a refusal to accept dialysis or a ventilator. However, doctors may be convinced that a particular intervention for a brief period of time will enable the patient to overcome a crisis and regain capacity along with a good quality of life. For this reason, some experts advise against articulating very specific preferences in advance directives. Instead, they recommend appointing an agent who will be familiar with the patient's general wishes but maintain broad discretion to make decisions on a case-by-case basis.[39]

Precedent Autonomy

Some clinicians may assert philosophical objections to following advance directive instructions for care limitation if the principal has developed dementia but seems to be living a contented life in this condition. The key question in the precedent autonomy debate is "Does an individual's request that simple life-sustaining treatment be avoided if he becomes demented remain valid into that dementia, when he may show apparent preferences to the contrary?"[40] In other words, do we defer to the autonomy of a preincapacity "then self," or do we instead focus on the altered "now self" and attempt to determine his or her wishes?

Consider the following example. A woman has an advance directive that instructs that if she is diagnosed with Alzheimer's disease or some other form of dementia, she should no longer be given treatment for any serious or life-threatening condition. Specifically, she states:

> Should I become severely demented, I do not wish to have my life extended by technological means unless as the unintended result of palliative measures. I refuse any artificial feeding and hydration, since forgetting how to swallow provides an opportunity to die in dignity. Further, I refuse dialysis, mechanical ventilation, resuscitation, and any and all efforts to apply these technologies. Likewise, I refuse antibiotics since pneumonia is a friend. The moral challenge for loved ones is only to be present with me, and to pray for me. In the event that I am in pain, keep me comfortable as needed.[41]

After being diagnosed with Alzheimer's disease, the patient develops pneumonia and needs antibiotics. What complicates matters is that she appears to be "pleasantly demented," that is, generally cheerful and enjoying simple pleasures such as eating and watching television. Her doctors feel extremely uncomfortable about forgoing therapy and allowing her to die of a very treatable condition.

Scholars have engaged in vigorous debate as to whether it is ethical to follow the principal's advance directive in these circumstances. Bioethicist Rebecca Dresser argues that if patients are able to enjoy and participate in their lives, it is not necessarily unethical to ignore their prior directives.[42] Treatment decisions should focus on the patient's "experiential reality." Indeed, memory loss and significant psychological changes may create a new person whose connection to the prior self is attenuated. By contrast, Professor Ronald Dworkin steadfastly defends precedent autonomy and individuals' right to maintain coherent life narratives, including end-of-life directives.[43]

It is thus possible that hospital authorities will refuse to follow the advance directive of a dementia patient who appears to enjoy daily pleasures. This may be particularly true if family members disagree with the wishes articulated in the document and argue passionately for continued care. It may also be true if no loved ones are present to insist that doctors adhere to the document's instructions.

HOSPITAL ETHICS COMMITTEES

How are health care decisions made for incapacitated patients who have no proxies or regarding whom there is disagreement among doctors and/or family members? A good option is to turn to the ethics committee, which exists at most hospitals and some long-term care organizations.[44] Ethics committees are composed of diverse stakeholders, including clinicians (doctors, nurses, pharmacists) with various areas of expertise, social workers, chaplains, ethicists, lawyers, and community representatives. Ethics committees are available for consultations in individual patient cases at the request of medical staff members. Consultations are conducted either by one expert consultant or by a subcommittee of several members. The committee may need to mediate among family members with conflicting views or, in some instances, to make a decision on behalf of the patient in the absence of any relatives or friends who are willing to become decision makers.[45]

I have served as a member of a hospital ethics committee for many years and am impressed by its work. The monthly meetings include thoughtful debates about important hospital policy matters and particularly challenging patient cases. I have also participated in ethics consults, most often regarding either termination of treatment for the dying or approval of medical procedures for incapacitated patients without proxies. The subcommittee always meets at length with the treating physicians and nurses and is serious, compassionate, thorough, and committed to making the best decision possible under the circumstances.

DURABLE POWER OF ATTORNEY FOR PROPERTY AND FINANCES

Medical treatment choices are not the only decisions that need to be made for individuals who become cognitively incapacitated. Financial decisions can be equally difficult and important. I now turn to a discussion of safeguards that can be implemented to ensure that your wishes concerning money and finances will be carried out if you lose capacity.

All states have power of attorney laws that enable an adult with decision-making capacity (called a principal) to delegate authority to handle financial and property matters to another person (called the agent, proxy, or attorney-in-fact). Some powers of attorney are "durable" because they are designed to continue to be effective in the event that the principal loses decision-making capacity. In some states, powers of attorney are automatically durable, and in others, the text must specify that they are durable or else they expire if the principal becomes incapacitated. Durable powers of attorney are an important tool for planning for old age. The document can be written long before there is a need for any agent and can state explicitly that the agent becomes empowered only upon the principal's incapacity.[46]

In the absence of a durable power of attorney, individuals who have lost capacity and cannot manage their own financial affairs will need to have a guardian (also called a conservator) appointed by a court. Guardianship proceedings can be initiated by interested parties such as family members or state agencies, but they can be lengthy and expensive, often lasting several months. Furthermore, the court may appoint a guardian who would not be the incompetent individual's first choice. Judges will likely opt for close family members, but the incompetent person may have previously experienced conflict with the designated guardian or may have a friend or domestic partner whom he or she would have preferred to have as a guardian.[47]

The law does not require that a lawyer prepare the power of attorney, and many states have statutory forms available on the Internet. However, consulting a lawyer is advisable because a legal professional can help you tailor the document to your needs and preferences.[48] States have varying execution requirements that range from only a signature to notarization with witnesses.

Powers of attorney generally give the agent (the person taking over) authority over all financial matters, including receiving, depositing, and writing checks; paying bills; managing bank accounts, CDs, stocks, bonds, and other investments; and taking possession or selling any real estate or personal property. In addition, you can empower the agent to make gifts, to establish a trust, to have access to safe deposit boxes, to pay taxes, and to engage in litigation on your behalf.[49]

Many people worry about agents taking advantage of their position, and those worries are legitimate. The elderly are particularly vulnerable to financial abuse, losing close to $3 billion in 2010, and this figure encompasses only documented cases. Abuse instances are thought to be woefully underreported, perhaps in part because at least one-third of them are perpetrated by people well known to the victim: relatives, friends, neighbors, and paid caregivers.[50] A dishonest or unreliable agent with broad powers will have ample opportunity to engage in wrongdoing, even to the extent of destroying the financial future of the principal and the principal's family. It is critical to realize that the agent will not be continuously supervised by any legal authority.[51]

The law affords some protection in a minority of states. The Uniform Power of Attorney Act (UPOAA) is a model law (a proposed law that states should consider) that seeks to promote durable power of attorney use while deterring agent misconduct, and it was adopted by 13 states as of 2013.[52] The UPOAA provides protection for both good-faith acceptance of a power of attorney and refusal to honor it in cases of suspected abuse. Under the law, there are also consequences for a party's *unreasonable* refusal to honor a power of attorney. The statute further clarifies the agent's duties, including (1) acting in good faith within his or her granted scope of authority and consistent with the principal's expectations or best interest, (2) preserving the principal's estate plan, and (3) cooperating with the principal's health care power of attorney (discussed above). In addition, the law includes liability provisions applicable to agents guilty of malfeasance, and it authorizes judicial review of agents' conduct. Finally, it requires that principals who wish to grant agents authority to make decisions that could dissipate their property or alter their estate plan, such as by gifting large sums or creating trusts, do so explicitly in the power of attorney document.[53]

Individuals should carefully choose not only the person to be named as agent but also the degree of power the agent will have. It is also wise to name a successor agent who can take over if the first individual becomes unable or unwilling to serve. Experts also recommend the establishment of oversight mechanisms. The agent can be instructed to provide periodic reports to an attorney or financial adviser and to have copies of financial statements regularly sent to a trusted third party to ensure the agent's good-faith conduct.[54]

WILLS, TRUSTS, TRANSFER ON DEATH, AND OTHER ASSET DISTRIBUTION INSTRUCTIONS

Finally, you should think about what will happen to your money and valuables after your death. Will they be distributed in accordance with your intentions? How difficult will it be for your loved ones to inherit your assets? A variety of legal instruments and instructions can help ensure that your wishes are carried out and that your survivors face as few hurdles as possible during the estate distribution process.

Wills

Preparing a will should be on every middle-aged person's agenda, including those who are not wealthy. Individuals without a will have no input as to how their assets are to be divided after their death, and their estates' distribution will be governed entirely by state law. Generally, under state intestate succession laws, only spouses, registered domestic partners, and blood relatives inherit. If the deceased person was married and is survived by his or her spouse, the spouse usually receives the largest portion of the estate, and if there are no children, the surviving spouse often receives all the property. Other parties such as unmarried partners, friends, and charities get nothing, and more distant relatives inherit only if there is no surviving spouse or child. If no relatives can be found, the state will take all of the assets.[55] If this is not how you would want your assets distributed after your death, you should be sure to have a will.

Those composing wills should name a trusted person (such as a spouse) as executor of the estate. They should also name an alternate executor (e.g., a younger sibling) who can serve if the first individual becomes unable or unwilling to do so.

Individuals with uncomplicated finances may opt to use an online service such as LegalZoom or USLegal in order to prepare their wills.* These websites charge very modest fees for simple wills, which in 2015 were advertised as costing well under $100.

Attorneys, however, generally advise against using an online service for a document that is as important as a will. Attorneys may charge hourly or flat fees for basic wills, and the cost is often under $500. Online wills may not be sufficiently customized for individual needs, especially for those with children from prior marriages, children with special needs, spouses with dementia, and any number of other complicated personal circumstances. Furthermore, in the absence of professional oversight, mistakes made by "do-it-yourself" users, such as clicking the wrong box, will not be caught. Decisions made without an expert's assistance can have serious adverse consequences in both personal and financial terms. An article in *Forbes* magazine describes the following "common trap":

> Mom wants to provide equally for her three children. Shares in GE con-
> stitute a third of her estate. So she leaves the stock to one child and the
> rest of her assets to the other two. Several months before she dies, she
> sells the stock. The child who was supposed to get it receives nothing.[56]

Occasionally, parents whose children have different income levels decide to minimize the inheritance of the child who earns the most or to exclude that child from inheriting altogether. Yet, however justified the parents think their conduct is, it is acutely painful for the disinherited individual and causes long-term tension and resentment among the siblings. An experienced elder law attorney or estate planning lawyer would counsel against making this mistake.

Trusts

Some people may also benefit from establishing a trust and should consult an attorney to explore this option. Professor Leon Gabinet, who is a col-league and an expert in trusts and estates, told me that he would advise any-one who owns a house and has a few hundred thousand dollars in additional assets (e.g., mutual funds or property) to establish a trust. There are a vari-ety of different types of trusts, but a common choice is a revocable living

---

*Respectively at http://www.legalzoom.com and http://www.uslegalforms.com/wills /?auslf=buildawill.

trust, which is a mechanism to avoid the expense and lengthy proceedings of probate for assets in the trust. Because probate proceedings are public, avoiding probate has the added advantage of protecting the deceased person's privacy.

Property in a trust is titled in the name of the trust and is managed by the trustee in accordance with instructions in the trust document. The trustee can be the person who created the trust. However, if you will manage your own trust during your lifetime, you should name a successor trustee and alternate successor trustee to take over in case you become incapacitated or die. An alternate is necessary to ensure that someone can take over if the original person you named dies, becomes incapacitated, or is otherwise unavailable.

Wealthy individuals can use professional trust companies to serve as trustees, although the fees for such services can be high. You can revise or revoke your trust at any time as long as you have mental capacity. In order to avoid probate completely, you must transfer all of your property to the trust, and if this is done, the trust will substitute for a will. Another advantage of a trust is that it can help families avoid guardianship proceedings. If the person who established the trust becomes incapacitated, a named trustee will manage the trust, and no other individual needs to be appointed by the court to serve as guardian to take care of financial matters. When you establish your trust, you can provide very detailed instructions. For example, you can include a directive that allows payment for long-term in-home care but not for permanent care in a nursing home if you wish to avoid being moved to a nursing facility as long as your money lasts.[57]

Transfer on Death

Property that is not included in a trust can be protected from probate through "transfer-on-death" (TOD) designation. TOD allows you to name beneficiaries who will receive your assets upon your death without needing to go through probate.[58] Bank accounts can be set up as payable on death, and brokerage accounts and vehicles can be registered as TOD, using forms obtained from financial institutions and the Department of Motor Vehicles. You can also obtain a TOD deed for real estate in some states. As in the case of wills and trusts, it is prudent to name alternate beneficiaries and to consult an attorney as to whether TOD registration is appropriate for particular assets.

Other Instructions

In order to help your family handle your affairs after your death, you should prepare several other documents as well. Be sure to keep track of all your assets and think about who should receive them, whether it be loved ones or charitable organizations. In addition to a will, it is wise to create a list of all valuables, such as jewelry and cars, with instructions as to who should inherit them. Forgetting to do this can cause tension, bitterness, and rivalries among children or siblings who want the same items.

In addition, you should create a memorandum that explains where important financial documents and items can be found (e.g., drawers at home, a home safe, a bank safe deposit box). You should give this memo to your agent for financial matters and to his or her alternate.

Instructions are also needed concerning desired funeral and burial or cremation arrangements. Do not assume that your loved ones will want to decide what to do with your remains. In many cases, they will appreciate clear guidance at a time that is chaotic and traumatic for them. When I first asked my parents where they wanted to be buried after my mother's breast cancer diagnosis in 1994, my mother said that she wanted to be buried in Israel, near her parents, and my father said he wanted to be buried in California, near his family members and in a place in which he spent many happy years as a young man. Puzzled, I asked them, "So, you don't want to be buried together?" They replied, "No, of course we want to be buried together—that is our priority." It was clear that we would need many family discussions to work this out, and happily, we had almost 20 years in which to do so. Ultimately, they decided to be buried in Michigan, where they had resided for the past three decades.

The average funeral in 2014 cost $7,000 to 10,000, but costs can vary widely. For example, a high-end casket alone can cost $10,000.[59] Some people feel strongly about how their remains should be handled or what they want included in or excluded from their funeral ceremony (prayers, music, poems). Others prioritize saving their families money, especially if they have no life insurance policy. It is not a kindness to withhold instructions from your survivors concerning a matter that will be difficult under the best of circumstances and can cause significant turmoil and strife.

LEGAL PREPAREDNESS CHECKLIST

All individuals who want to have a say in how they will be treated if they become incapacitated and what will happen to their assets in case of incapacity or death should implement multiple levels of legal protection. What follows is a legal preparedness checklist:

- No single document is sufficient. You should have a will (and possibly a trust), a durable power of attorney for property and finances, a living will, a durable power of attorney for health care, and if desired, an anatomical gift form. The latter three forms may be combined into a single advance directive for health care if permitted under state law.

Those with a history of mental illness should also consider executing a separate advance directive for mental health treatment.

- If an attorney will not be helping you prepare your documents, consult other sources. The websites LegalZoom and USLegal provide users with various legal forms that can be filled out. Likewise, the American Bar Association Commission on Law and Aging provides a useful resource for those interested in preparing advance directives. It is called the *Consumer's Tool Kit for Health Care Advance Planning* and is available on the Internet.[60]

- You should check all personal legal documents, including wills, every five years to ensure that they are still accurate and reflect your wishes. In addition, you should revisit them anytime an important life event occurs, such as divorce, death of an immediate family member, or a significant change in health status, because these may necessitate modifications to the documents' text.[61]

- If you move to a different state, you should execute a new advance directive that conforms to its laws. Similarly, if you spend significant time in more than one state, for example, you winter in Florida or Arizona but live elsewhere the rest of the year, you should have advance directives for each of the states in which you live.[62]

- It is also important for you to remain in close touch with your proxies for health care and property to ensure that they continue to be available, trustworthy, and willing to follow instructions. In some cases, for example, health care proxies may change their minds about end-of-life issues and may grow uncomfortable rejecting aggressive care or requesting its withdrawal. If this occurs and is inconsistent with your wishes, you should execute a new advance directive and name a different agent. You should also verify that your agent fully understands your wishes and attitudes about medical interventions in various circumstances so that he or she can make appropriate decisions in the absence of explicit instructions in the advance directive.

- You should have repeated discussions about your care preferences in case of dementia both with your health care proxy and with others who are likely to be involved in future decisions about your care. Such conversations might provide sufficient evidence to overcome clinicians' and other loved ones' concerns about precedent autonomy and a "now self" whose wishes or interests are different from those of the "then self."

- Making sure that the people who will determine your care in case you become incapacitated know that you have an advance directive is of critical importance. To this end, you should not only retain copies of the documentation, but also give copies to your proxies and alternates, treating physicians, and hospitals and nursing home at which you receive care. Advance directive wallet cards are also available.[63]

- Take advantage of electronic means that can enhance the likelihood that your advance directive will be seen and followed by appropriate medical personnel. Ask your doctors if they have posted a copy of your advance directive in your medical record. Some electronic health records (EHR) have an alert that indicates the presence of an advance directive. If you have treating physicians at different facilities with different EHR systems, give a copy to each doctor so that the separate EHRs each contain a copy of the document. You will need to ask doctors in different medical practices whether they need their own copy of your advance directive. Several private organizations offer advance directive registries, and some states* have established registries as well. Private organizations, such as DocuBank, U.S. Living Will Registry, and others, store advance directives with unique registration numbers. They provide customers with wallet cards and labels for their driver's licenses and insurance cards that list their registration numbers. Health care providers who know the registration number (or patient's social security number) can contact the registry and request a copy of the document.[64]
- If you will receive care at a hospital either as an inpatient or an outpatient, take your advance directive with you and make sure it is entered into the hospital's EMR system.

Does legal preparedness make a difference? The answer is yes. According to a large study published in the *New England Journal of Medicine*, patients with advance directives generally received end-of-life care that was consistent with their treatment preferences. Thus, if competently prepared and appropriately distributed, living wills and durable power of attorney for health care documents significantly impact decision-making outcomes and help promote treatment plans that reflect patients' wishes.[65] If you care about what happens to your money and your medical treatment in the event of your incapacity and you have specific wishes regarding how your property should be distributed upon your death, then preparing the documents described in this chapter is well worth the time and effort.

---

*The states include Arizona, California, Idaho, Louisiana, Montana, Nevada, North Carolina, Vermont, and Virginia.

5

Driving While Elderly

Not long ago, my local newspaper, *The Cleveland Plain Dealer*, featured a large photograph of a frail, elderly woman sitting at a table in a courtroom with her head bent, her eyes closed, and her folded hands pressed against her forehead. The woman looked devastated, and the reason became clear as soon as I read the story's headline: "Driver in Fatal Hit-Skip Avoids Prison Time."[1] The 81-year-old driver had caused the death of a 13-year-old boy, perhaps because a prescription drug had impaired her faculties. Although she avoided prison, she was required to pay considerable restitution to the boy's family, will be under house arrest for five years, and will likely be tormented by guilt to the end of her days.

This is not a unique story. Several similar tragedies have received extensive media coverage. In 2012, a 100-year-old man in Los Angeles backed his Cadillac into a crowd by an elementary school, hitting 11 and seriously injuring four children.[2] Years earlier, an 86-year-old driver lost control of his car and sped through a farmers market, killing nine and hurting more than 50 people.[3]

My own neighborhood in Cleveland is home to many seniors. In the past few years, three of the businesses that my husband and I frequent suddenly had their front windows boarded up. In each instance, we were told that an elderly driver had hit the accelerator rather than the brakes when trying to park directly in front of the store or restaurant. In one case, a few days after the accident, the large dumpster into which the owners threw items damaged in the accident was also hit. It turned out that the "culprit" was the very same driver.

Many people with disabilities, including those who are elderly, reach a point at which they should voluntarily refrain from getting behind the wheel because of physical or cognitive impairments. Refusing to stop driving at the appropriate time is socially irresponsible and potentially catastrophic. At worst, it can lead to injury or death of the elderly driver or another party, and in some instances, will create significant financial difficulties for one's heirs. For example, an elderly acquaintance had a minor car accident two months before she died of unrelated causes. The other driver claimed that she had suffered a neck injury that caused her to endure a long-term disability, to undergo surgery, and to be unable to continue working in her physically demanding profession. She sued both the insurer and the elderly driver's estate, and the family could not distribute the estate assets until the matter was resolved.

Admittedly, however, the end of driving can lead to a demoralizing loss of autonomy, a diminishing sense of self-worth, and a need for major lifestyle adjustments. It can also inhibit social interaction and lead to a significant deterioration in quality of life. Adequate transportation may be essential to continued social engagement, participation in cultural, religious, and recreational activities, access to goods and services including medical care, and a sense of belonging to your community.[4] In many locations, public transportation is poor to nonexistent. A report written by Transportation for America estimated that by 2015, more than 15.5 million older Americans will face poor transit access.[5] Seniors' reluctance to stop driving is thus often understandable and can become a major source of conflict for families. Learning how to have constructive conversations about driving with the elderly, finding transportation alternatives, and acknowledging that you may not be able to drive forever are important steps in planning for your old age and that of loved ones.

The Federal Highway Administration estimated that 23.1 million individuals 70 and older had licenses in 2012. Thus, approximately 79 percent of those in the 70 and up population still have licenses, constituting 11 percent of all drivers.[6] In fact, some people continue to drive even after they reach the age of 100; in 2013, Florida reported it had 455 licensed drivers who were 100 or older.[7]

Does empirical evidence support the claim that elderly drivers pose more of a risk to public safety than others? A number of studies have probed this question, and the answer appears to be only a weak yes.

DRIVING AND COLLISION STATISTICS

To what extent do we really need to worry that elderly drivers are a hazard on the road? The data are more reassuring than I expected.

In 2012, 4,079 people ages 70 and older died in auto accidents.[8] The Centers for Disease Control and Prevention (CDC) asserts that, per mile traveled, fatal accident rates increase beginning at age 75, and the rate accelerates after age 80, with those 85 and older facing the highest risk of dying while behind the wheel.[9] However, the fact that deaths are more common among older drivers who have accidents is largely attributable to their frailty.[10] People who are frail are more likely to die of accident-related injuries than younger, sturdier individuals. Consequently, these fatal accidents are fatal mostly for the older drivers themselves and their elderly passengers.

In defense of older drivers, those who are 75 or older kill fewer pedestrians, bicyclists, motorcyclists, and occupants of other cars than do drivers in the age group of 30 to 59, and teenagers pose a greater risk than any other group.[11] In addition, research shows that fatality rates for all drivers decreased between 1998 and 2012, but the decline, measured at 31 percent, was particularly pronounced for those who were 70 and older.[12]

Although the youngest drivers are the most likely to have accidents, seniors have the second highest rate of involvement in collisions per mile driven. Insurance claims for property damage and collisions increase after age 65.[13]

Regardless of the statistics, if you live to be old enough, there may well come a time when you have to stop driving. Will the government tell you when that time has come? Do state authorities offer clear guidance?

STATE REGULATION

When I began conducting research for this chapter, I assumed that the states had implemented regulatory safeguards designed to keep unsafe elderly drivers off the roads. These would be a logical parallel to the prohibition on driving by those who are too young and on the requirement of road tests before issuance of the first license. I knew that there were gaps in state regulations because several of my elderly acquaintances have received no more than a traffic ticket even after driving their cars into fire hydrants or parked vehicles. One was easily able to renew her driver's license at 92, despite using a walker, which should have raised questions about her ability to control the car pedals with her legs. Nevertheless, I had imagined that regulation in this area was more robust than it is, and I was surprised by how little certainty there is about what interventions are effective.

Special provisions for older drivers have been enacted by 30 states and the District of Columbia, but these are generally limited to increased renewal frequency, renewal in person, and vision tests. Only the District of Columbia and Nevada require a medical certification after age 70, and only Illinois requires a road test for those 75 or older. To check the state license renewal

requirements for older drivers in your state, you may refer to a chart com-
piled by the Insurance Institute for Highway Safety, which can be found on
its website.[14]

The absence of more aggressive regulation may be due in part to concerns
about age discrimination. If states implemented a rule that made renewal
much more difficult after a certain age, they could be accused of violating
the constitutional principle of equal protection of the law. Opponents could
argue that younger people are not subject to the same requirements even if
they have disabilities that could potentially affect their driving ability, but
older individuals face automatic renewal hurdles regardless of their health
status.

In truth, there is little evidence that strict regulations that would limit
driving by the elderly would make the roads safer. California pilot tested
a three-tier evaluation for driver's license renewal by all applicants, which
required that those who failed the first two tiers take an on-road test. The
first-tier screening consisted of a brief memory recall test, two vision tests,
and the tester's observation of any visible physical limitations. The second tier
consisted of a written test of driving knowledge and a perceptual response
test designed to identify limitations in perception and cognition that are relevant to driving.[15] The state found only weak indications that the program
reduced at-fault collisions with injuries or fatalities. A study in Maryland,
however, revealed that individuals who were 78 and older and performed
poorly on certain cognitive tests were twice as likely as other drivers to cause
crashes.[16] Although some literature supports the implementation of vision
tests for older license applicants, road tests face more opposition because they
are costly and burdensome, and experts have argued that there is an insufficient basis for requiring them routinely for any age group.[17] Researchers
have also found that states with special requirements for elderly drivers had
a 17 percent lower fatality rate per licensed driver among those 85 and older
but no reduction when the study population was expanded to 65 and older.
Other studies found that various regulatory interventions had no impact at
all.[18] Research results are thus confusing and inconsistent. It is noteworthy,
however, that there is evidence that stringent state licensing requirements can
induce drivers to decide to reduce or stop driving of their own accord, presumably because they wish to avoid undergoing a rigorous renewal process.[19]

While AAA, AARP, and others offer educational courses for older drivers,
the Insurance Institute for Highway Safety concludes that "[t]here is little evidence of safety benefits from education courses for older drivers."[20] This is perhaps because the classes are voluntary and thus attract a self-selected group of
seniors who are especially conscientious. Those who enroll are already among
the safest drivers and the least likely to be involved in collisions.

Perhaps most troubling is the lack of structured reporting mechanisms
for identifying at-risk drivers and for addressing the dangers they pose. Only

eight states mandate that physicians report at-risk drivers to state authorities,[21] although all states permit doctors to do so. The states vary as to whether they accept reports from family members, friends, or anonymous sources and as to how such reports are to be submitted (e.g., by letter, form, or e-mail).[22] In addition, fewer than half the states are known to train law enforcement officers to identify and report medically at-risk drivers.[23] This training gap is particularly disturbing. A police officer who is called to the scene of an accident and simply tickets an elderly driver who seems confused or has a history of multiple recent collisions may endanger public safety by failing to alert state authorities and to request follow-up action.

Reliance on family and friends as the primary source of information about seniors who should not be driving is dubious at best. Those who are close to the elderly individual may not be willing to jeopardize their relationship with him or her by informing authorities of their concerns. Many states do not provide confidentiality protection for such reports. At the same time, many elderly people would know who contacted the authorities because they had prior confrontations about driving with these individuals. Several of my acquaintances have tried threatening their loved ones with a report to authorities and have promptly been told they would never be spoken to again if that happened.

If the state is notified of an at-risk driver, it may intervene in a variety of ways. State authorities will likely first consult the state's medical advisory board (if one exists), the driver's own physician, or another health care provider. Short of revoking the elderly person's license, the state may impose driving restrictions, such as prohibiting driving on high-speed roads, at night, or outside a certain area.[24] Although older drivers may initially feel resentful, these limitations can actually enable seniors to remain independent and continue driving safely for a significant period of time.[25]

One encouraging research finding is that older drivers engage in some degree of self-regulation, even without state-imposed constraints. They are more likely than others to wear seatbelts, to limit driving in bad weather and after dark, to drive short distances, and to drive sober.[26] In 2008, drivers who were 70 and older drove an average of 45 percent fewer miles than drivers in the 35 to 54 age group.[27]

As the population ages, further research will hopefully be done to determine which, if any, interventions are effective. In 2014, Canada's Ministry of Transportation took an interesting approach in Ontario, requiring the following of drivers 80 and older: (1) a vision test, (2) in-class group education, (3) a review of the driver's record, and (4) two exercises consisting of drawing the hands of a clock to 11:10 and crossing out each "H" from rows of letters in order to test basic competencies.[28] If the outcomes of this experiment are studied after a couple of years, perhaps they will be illuminating for U.S. policymakers as well.

KNOWING WHEN TO STOP DRIVING AND MAKING IT HAPPEN

Everyone must accept that there may come a time when driving will no longer be a safe activity. It may become too dangerous because of physical disabilities, mental impairments, or the use of prescription drugs whose side effects impact wakefulness, reaction time, and mental acuity. AAA offers an Internet resource called Roadwise rx* that allows individuals who are taking prescription drugs to search for medication interactions, food interactions, and driver warnings. Discussions with prescribing physicians about the impact of new medications on driving ability are also advisable.

The Signs of Danger

How do you know when you or a loved one should consider turning in your driver's license? The AARP lists these signs:

- Health or medication changes
- Getting lost in familiar areas
- Car crashes
- Near misses
- Scrapes on the car
- Swerving or driving over curbs
- Difficulty with left turns
- Driving at inappropriate speeds
- Incorrect signaling
- Failure to notice traffic signs or stop at red lights
- Mixing up the gas and brake pedals
- Confusion at highway exits.[29]

If you are unsure about whether you or a loved one can continue to drive safely, you can get a comprehensive driving evaluation from an occupational therapist. These evaluations are administered at rehabilitation centers, hospitals, and Veterans' Administration Medical Centers and generally cost $200 to $500. Evaluators will not only determine whether it is appropriate for the individual to drive, but will provide advice regarding limitations (e.g., nighttime driving) or equipment (e.g., wide range mirrors) that should be adopted to promote safe driving.

---

*Available at http://www.roadwiserx.com/.

Having the Conversation

Confronting elderly loved ones who are not inclined to stop driving despite danger signs can be excruciatingly difficult. In my own family, such conversations have been painful. "You have been a generous, kind, hard-working person your entire life. Why are you courting tragedy now? How would you like to live your remaining years knowing that you have injured or even killed another human being because you won't face reality about your driving abilities?" Apparently, this is not an ideal approach!

The AARP provides the following tips to help you prepare for discussions with elderly drivers about their driving future:

- Find several opportunities to be a passenger in the older driver's car to observe his or her driving skills and habits.
- Build consensus among family and friends before approaching the elderly driver about the matter.
- Select the right person to be the messenger and do not involve the police.
- Choose the right time. Do not have upsetting conversations about the elderly person's ability to drive while he or she is behind the wheel.
- Be prepared to have multiple conversations before achieving your goal. Build up from casual chats to more serious, action-oriented discussions.
- When you have the conversation, listen to the elderly driver, ask questions about his or her feelings, and validate any concerns about what losing the freedom to drive will mean.
- Ask elderly drivers what their own thoughts are about their driving abilities.
- Emphasize that you care about the safety of the driver, passengers, and the public.
- Present concrete examples of driving mistakes based on your observations rather than discussing assumptions based on the driver's age or complaints you have heard from others.[30]

FINDING TRANSPORTATION RESOURCES

Living in a retirement community (as discussed in Chapter 2) is one way to minimize the impact of surrendering your driver's license. Such communities may provide many on-campus amenities that reduce the need for a car. They may also offer routine and individually arranged transportation to various off-campus destinations, such as medical offices, grocery stores, and cultural events. Those living in other residential settings may be able to ask nearby friends or relatives to carpool for errands and entertainment and to assist with other transportation needs.

Many communities have supplemental transportation programs for the elderly.[31] These programs use volunteers or charge a minimal fee per ride. Residents can obtain information about local programs by calling their city hall. AAA also has a tool on its website that enables users to search for alternative transportation programs.* Advocates have urged that government offices and aging-oriented organizations develop hotlines, directories, marketing information, and educational programs to inform the public about local transportation options. The available choices, however, are generally limited by financial and staffing constraints, and seniors may find them less than ideal in terms of convenience and responsiveness to their needs.[32]

Another option is to hire aides who will do the driving or run errands for elderly clients. These can be retained by contacting local home care agencies or searching online. For example, an Internet resource called Care.com contains listings of individuals offering a variety of services, ranging from babysitting to elder care. Care.com verifies the identity of those advertising their services and can be asked to conduct full background checks. My family posted an ad on Craigslist when we needed someone to help my father with driving and other tasks. We then used the Internet service called Intelius to conduct a background check on the successful applicant prior to hiring him. Those who are active in a religious community may also ask their clergy if they can recommend responsible individuals who would like to work as occasional drivers for elderly community members.

In addition, there are a variety of ways to reduce the number of errands you have to run. Many grocery stores and restaurants offer delivery services. A great deal of shopping can also be accomplished through the Internet at home. Thus, seniors can balance the psychological benefits of leaving the house and mingling with others against the need for convenience and reduced access to transportation.

THE AID OF TECHNOLOGY

With emerging improvements in technology, older drivers may be able to extend their safe driving years. Many driver assistance systems have already been developed and are increasingly common in 21st-century vehicles. These include navigation systems, park distance information, lane departure warnings, automated emergency braking, automated headlights, and pedestrian detection.[33] Rear backup cameras provide drivers with a view of what is behind the car when it is in reverse and help them judge distances and back up safely.[34] A feature called "adaptive cruise control" automatically adjusts the

---

*Available at http://seniordriving.aaa.com/map.

speed of a car on cruise control when the speed of the car ahead of it changes in order to maintain a specified distance between the two vehicles.[35] Traffic jam assist uses sensors and software that adjust speed and handle braking and steering in heavy traffic that moves at up to 37 miles per hour.[36] The pre-safe brake feature causes the car to stop if a pedestrian is detected and the driver fails to step on the brake pedal.[37]

Some experts even predict that in a couple of decades, we will have autonomous vehicles in which all driving functions are automated at all times.[38] Such technology, however, still faces significant technological barriers and may be hindered by concerns about legal liability, insurance regulation, and public acceptance.[39]

Older car buyers should carefully investigate vehicle safety features and consider them central to their purchasing decisions. More important, as baby boomers age, we cannot ignore the likelihood that we will have to stop driving altogether in our later years. The availability of convenient and affordable transportation alternatives should be a factor in selecting retirement homes and communities.

DRIVING PREPAREDNESS CHECKLIST

- Be committed to recognizing when it is unsafe for you to drive and to stop of your own accord at the appropriate time.
- Be attuned to signs that you or your loved one is having driving difficulties.
- Seek a comprehensive driving evaluation if there is uncertainty about driving abilities.
- Approach conversations with older drivers carefully. Be sensitive to their feelings and present them with evidence of specific driving problems.
- Keep transportation needs in mind when selecting a retirement community.
- Investigate transportation options before asking a loved one to stop driving.
- As you age, pay special attention to safety features and safety-oriented technology when purchasing automobiles.

6

Coordinated Care: Treating the Patient, not Diseases

In April 2012, a little over a year before she died, something terrible happened to my mother. Eema, as we called her in Hebrew, had just returned from a trip to Israel with my sister, where they attended a young cousin's wedding. Seemingly overnight, Eema transformed from being a relatively active, alert 83-year-old to behaving as though she had advanced dementia. When she talked, she made no sense, and frequently, she was completely uncommunicative. She slept for much of the day and often sat in front of the television with a blank stare when she was awake. She showed little interest in eating and drinking and lost weight rapidly. The local hospital admitted Eema for a couple of days and then transferred her to a psychiatric ward elsewhere. My sister who lives in the same city soon demanded that Eema be released because her mental state deteriorated even further.

What had happened? Eema's treating physicians provided no answers. My three sisters and I decided to take matters into our own hands. We spent countless hours doing Internet searches, calling every acquaintance who was a medical professional, and e-mailing our findings to each other. We ultimately determined that the problem was severe drug interactions. Eema had been taking about a dozen medications, and then one more was added—an antidepressant that was prescribed after my father reported to their doctor that she seemed somewhat lethargic and glum. The internist vaguely told Eema that it was another pill to help her sleep, because he knew she would refuse any psychiatric intervention and would resist being labeled as clinically depressed. The drastic change in her demeanor came days after she began taking the new drug.

The hospital and several doctors dismissed the possibility that the small dose of the antidepressant had led to instantaneous dementia. Nevertheless, we decided on our own to take Eema off the medication, first reducing the dose to half, but quickly eliminating it completely when the half-dose seemed to exacerbate her confusion. There was some improvement, but not a dramatic one. Upon learning about the phenomenon of drug-induced delirium, we urged my sister to take Eema to the emergency room again. Testing revealed that Eema's blood had dangerously high levels of digoxin, a heart medication. When this medication's level was stabilized, there was further improvement, but Eema was still far from her old self. We continued our research, studying the side effects of all of her drugs and identifying several that were listed as potentially impacting cognitive functioning. Each of Eema's specialists argued against eliminating any drugs that he had prescribed, but we persisted, and one by one all medications that were not clearly medically necessary at her age were discontinued, until she was down to five instead of 12 prescriptions. Miraculously, Eema regained her full mental capacities. She had no memory of a two-month period spanning from mid-April to mid-June 2012.

Is this story unique? Apparently not. Richard Russo's book *Elsewhere: A Memoir* contains an account of a similar episode involving his mother. One day she was fine. Then the next morning he found her disheveled, confused, and incoherent, like "the madwoman in the attic, straight out of *Jane Eyre*." Once hospitalized, the author's mother was taken off all of her medications except for blood pressure pills, and I was not surprised to read that she "returned to the old normal" after four days.[1]

Researchers have confirmed that overprescription is a common medical error. ProPublica* conducted an analysis of Medicare prescription records from the years 2007 to 2010 and found that "some doctors and other health professionals across the country prescribe large quantities of drugs that are potentially harmful, disorienting or addictive for their patients."[2] Data from the Centers for Disease Control and Prevention suggest that nearly half of Americans are taking at least one prescription drug, one in five takes three, and over 10 percent take five or more prescription medications.[3] The three most commonly prescribed drugs are antibiotics, antidepressants, and painkillers.[4] In a book called *Overtreated: Why Too Much Medicine Is Making Us*

---

*ProPublica describes itself as "an independent, non-profit newsroom that produces investigative journalism in the public interest." Accessed October 20, 2014, http://www.propublica.org/about/.

Sicker and Poorer, Shannon Brownlee argues that the drug and device industries have persuaded "both patients and doctors that we're sicker than we really are, and that the path to wellness lies with medical intervention: with a pill, an operation, or a test." Thus these industries have transformed us "into a nation of the worried well."[5]

How could incidents such as the one endured by Eema be avoided? Medical oversight by a skilled internist or geriatric specialist who can coordinate the care of a patient with multiple medical problems may be the most promising answer. In addition, patients must learn to be active members of their own medical teams and to seek the support and counsel of advocates who can assist them with navigating the complexities of medical care.

Although middle-aged individuals will not themselves visit geriatricians, old-age preparedness requires familiarity with this specialty. In addition, those with aging loved ones whose medical problems are becoming more numerous and serious may seek the involvement of a geriatrician in order to improve care coordination.

THE PRACTICE OF GERIATRICS

Geriatricians are physicians with special training in evaluating and managing the care needs of older adults. Treating this population requires expertise not only in internal medicine, but also in neurology, psychiatry, rehabilitative medicine, and other specialties. Elderly patients commonly suffer from multiple medical conditions, and geriatricians often must address some combination of dementia, depression, mobility impairments, incontinence, chronic pain, sensory limitations, and end-of-life decision making.[6]

Geriatricians generally work with interdisciplinary teams to provide elderly patients with comprehensive care. They may partner with nurses, physician assistants, social workers, pharmacists, nutritionists, physical and occupational therapists, speech and hearing specialists, and geriatric psychiatrists.[7] Mental health services are often particularly important for elderly patients. The National Alliance on Mental Illness estimates that close to 20 percent of seniors suffer from depression, and their illness often goes untreated.[8]

One of the most important benefits geriatricians can provide to their patients is coordination of overall care. The elderly often see a number of different specialists, including cardiologists, oncologists, rheumatologists, endocrinologists, and others. According to an article in the *Journal of the American Geriatrics Society,* in 2008 patients 75 years of age and older saw specialists more often than generalist physicians (56 percent of the time).[9] A different study estimated that one-third of elderly patients saw specialists but not primary care physicians and that the average number of different specialists whom they saw was four.[10] Care of the elderly can thus be fragmented, with each specialist focusing only on complaints that fall within his or her area of expertise and providing aggressive treatment for those problems.

Patients who suffer from chronic pain may be particularly persistent in pursuing the care of specialists and experimenting with new drugs and treatments. A considerable segment of the elderly population is included among chronic pain patients—as many as 17.5 million elderly individuals report recurring pain,[11] most commonly in the neck, back, knees, or legs.[12]

Although responsible doctors generally ask patients to report what other medications they are taking, patients may provide incomplete accounts (especially those with memory impairments), and specialists may check only for well-established drug interactions involving pairs of drugs rather than combinations of three or more medications. Without a geriatric expert, there may be nobody who will ask whether patients are taking too many drugs, whether the full combination of drugs is causing them harm, or whether their most pressing problems are being addressed.

Both my mother and mother-in-law visited geriatricians for comprehensive workups. Our families were impressed with the attention both received at their initial visits. In each case, the appointment began with a social worker who asked questions about their living situations, social support, and ability to perform activities of daily living and then conducted cognitive testing. The geriatric physicians then spent a full hour taking a thorough medical history, reviewing all available documentation, and paying special attention to all the medications they were taking. After ordering blood tests, follow-up appointments were scheduled for the next month.

Dr. Atul Gawande, a surgeon and journalist, writes the following about geriatric care:

> Most of us in medicine . . . don't know how to think about decline. We're good at addressing specific, individual problems: colon cancer, high blood pressure, arthritic knees. Give us a disease, and we can do something about it. But give us an elderly woman with colon cancer, high blood pressure, arthritic knees, and various other ailments besides—an elderly woman at risk of losing the life she enjoys—and we are not sure what to do.[13]

Dr. Gawande published an article in the *New Yorker* in 2007 in which he described sitting in on one patient's appointment at his hospital's geriatrics clinic. To his surprise, the geriatrician paid particular attention to the patient's feet. A primary concern, the doctor explained, is an elderly person's risk of falling, and the condition of a patient's feet is highly relevant (poor balance, taking more than four prescription drugs, and muscle weakness also increase the probability of falling). At the end of the visit, the doctor formulated two key recommendations: the woman was to obtain regular care from a podiatrist and to increase her calorie intake.[14]

Gawande notes that geriatricians do not perform "high-tech medicine." Instead, they simplify medications and try to ensure that arthritis is controlled, feet are in acceptable shape, and nutritious meals are eaten. They also investigate whether the patient is socially isolated or living in a home that is unsafe. Gawande reports that research findings indicate that patients under the care of a geriatrics team are significantly less likely than other elderly people to become disabled or depressed or to require home health services.[15]

THE SHORTAGE OF GERIATRICIANS

Unfortunately, the United States faces a grave shortage of geriatricians, and thus you may not be able to find a geriatrician for your relatives or yourself when you need one. As of March 2011, there were 7,162 certified geriatricians nationwide,[16] and fewer than 350 physicians entered geriatric medicine fellowships each year.[17] These figures represent a more than 20 percent decrease in the number of geriatricians since 2000.[18] The shortage extends to geriatric medical specialties as well. For example, geriatric psychiatrists are difficult to locate. According to one source, there are only 1,700 board-certified geriatric psychiatrists practicing in the United States, that is, one for every 23,000 seniors.[19] Likewise, by 2005, approximately 200 dentists had received postdoctoral training in geriatric dentistry, although experts estimate that 7,000 dentists with geriatric training are needed to treat the elderly in this country.[20] The shortage of geriatricians is particularly acute in rural areas.[21]

When my parents, in their mid-eighties, finally sought the care of a geriatrician in East Lansing, Michigan, they learned that there was only one geriatric medicine practice in the area. Those clinicians were so overwhelmed that they declined to accept new patients. Instead, my mother turned to a geriatrics practice in Ann Arbor, which is more than an hour away.

And matters are likely to get worse as baby boomers age. Some commentators predict that in order to meet the needs of our rapidly growing population of seniors, the United States should produce 36,000 new geriatricians by 2030.[22] But this increase is very unlikely to materialize.

Why can't medical schools produce more geriatricians so that at least younger baby boomers can be reassured that our needs will be met? Geriatrics has been a certified specialty for approximately 20 years. Among the 141 accredited medical schools in the United States, 105 feature identifiable geriatric academic programs,[23] but only 14 boast geriatrics departments.[24] In a 2007 survey of graduating medical students, only 23 percent of respondents indicated that they "strongly agreed that they were exposed to expert geriatric care."[25] Worse yet, academic geriatrics programs may face a wave of departures in the near future. In 2010, 39 percent of program directors indicated that they planned to leave their leadership positions by 2015.[26]

A significant barrier to entry into the field of geriatrics is a comparatively low earning potential, which likely concerns medical students who are encumbered by significant educational debt. Geriatricians are reimbursed largely by Medicare. In 2010, the median salary of geriatricians in private practice was $183,523, whereas that of a neurologist was $249,867.[27]

PLANNING FOR MEDICAL CARE IN OLD AGE

As noted above, geriatricians treat only elderly individuals, and thus, even the most dedicated planners for old age cannot obtain care from a geriatric specialist earlier in life. Nevertheless, forming good habits regarding medical care in middle age is essential to good health later in life.

Finding a Doctor

Those of us who have experienced significant health problems at a relatively young age are often particularly careful about checkups and preventive care. Nevertheless, by age 50, everyone should be diligent about following medical guidelines regarding checkups and preventive care. To this end, middle-aged individuals should have primary care physicians who are familiar with their medical histories and can coordinate their care if they develop multiple medical ailments. Those with good internists who know them well and with whom they are comfortable will not need to switch to a geriatrician in old age. As noted by several experts "[t]he importance of a primary care physician in the care of all conditions, except those that are highly complex or rare, is increasingly recognized."[28]

Unfortunately, even finding an internist who accepts new patients and who is available and attentive may be easier said than done. Our country is experiencing not only a shortage of geriatricians, but also a significant dearth of primary care physicians. The AARP reports that we have 16,000 fewer primary care physicians than we need, and this shortfall is likely attributable to the large discrepancy between the salaries of primary care physicians and those of other specialists.[29] Recently, only about 7 percent of medical school graduates have been choosing primary care careers.[30] Furthermore, about one-quarter of primary care physicians are nearing retirement age themselves, which may exacerbate the shortage in the near future.[31]

Thus, identifying and selecting a good internist can be difficult work in and of itself. Friends and acquaintances are often a trustworthy source of information, so you should not hesitate to ask for recommendations. Patient reviews on the Internet are a more dubious source. Frequently, there are only a handful of comments, so they are not necessarily representative of most patients' experiences. Moreover, there is no way to verify that those who post comments anonymously are actually the doctors' patients rather than family members, friends, competitors, or others with a personal agenda.

You should look for doctors whose patient population includes many elderly people, because they are more likely to be familiar with health problems commonly found in this age group. You may also want to find a practice that employs nurse practitioners or physician assistants because such practices may provide more accessibility and responsiveness to patients. Nurse practitioners and physician assistants are highly trained professionals and sometimes receive special instruction in geriatric matters.[32] Because they are paid lower salaries and bill at lower rates than physicians, they are often the ones who spend extensive time interacting with patients while the doctor moves quickly from one exam room to another. Patients may find that nurse practitioners and physician assistants take time to answer questions thoroughly either in person or by phone and to provide reassuring explanations. Thus, access to these health care professionals may significantly enhance patients' medical experiences.

Many seniors will never see a geriatrician either because they cannot find one or because their medical problems are well handled by their internists. Those with multiple and complex conditions, however, should make a special effort to obtain regular care from a geriatric expert, or, at the very least, to visit a geriatrician for a onetime thorough exam and evaluation. Such a consultation can enable elderly people (or relatives who accompany them) to determine whether they are receiving appropriate care from their internists or whether they need to switch doctors or see specialists.

It is possible that electronic health records (EHRs), which are being adopted by most medical practices, will facilitate care coordination for elderly patients. EHR systems should help physicians check for drug interactions, allergies, and medical histories and should provide decision support in the form of alerts and reminders about dosages, screening tests, and treatment protocols that can be critical to patient safety.

However, contemporary EHRs have many limitations. Decision support is sometimes flawed, providing incorrect information or alerts that are irrelevant and distracting to physicians. Voluminous records are tough to navigate and make it difficult for busy clinicians to review the essential components of a patient's medical history quickly and efficiently. Furthermore, many patients visit doctors at different facilities or health networks whose EHR systems are not interoperable so that the patients' records remain fragmented. Pieces of the record are housed in different medical practices and cannot be put together into an all-inclusive file. Moreover, many doctors complain that extensive data entry requirements take time away from examining and listening to the patient and thinking deeply about diagnosis and treatment. Some also find that the computer's presence disrupts the doctor–patient relationship because patients become frustrated that the doctor is paying more attention to the computer than to them at the bedside or in the exam room.[33] Until significant technological improvements are achieved, EHR systems on their own are unlikely to go far enough to address the care coordination needs of elderly patients.

Concierge Medicine

Concierge medicine* is an option for individuals who are financially comfortable. Under this model, primary care physicians charge annual out-of-pocket fees and can thus afford to see fewer patients so that they can dedicate more time to them. The fees average $1,500 but can be as large as $15,000. In return, concierge doctors promise patients same-day or next-day care, thorough preventive medical services, and 24-hour-a-day access through cell phones and e-mail so that they can be contacted at anytime from anywhere in the country or the world.[34]

Concierge doctors have adopted a variety of charge structures. Some physicians charge only an annual fee, while others require both an annual fee and payment for individual office visits. Some bill insurance companies; some prefer to avoid the administrative burdens of billing insurers; and still others continue to run regular primary care practices, setting aside a few hours a day for their retainer-based patients.[35]

In early 2013, there were 5,000 to 5,500 concierge physicians in the United States out of about 240,000 primary care physicians providing direct patient care. In 2014, the number may have risen to 12,000.[36] Further research is needed as to how satisfied patients are with their services and whether they have better health outcomes. A major advantage is that such doctors can limit their patient intake to an average of 350, compared to 1,475 that are accepted by a typical primary care physician.[37] Concierge doctors can provide patients with far more accessibility, attentiveness, and services than ordinary primary care physicians with much busier practices.

Being a Member of Your Own Medical Team

On October 15, 2013, my husband, at the age of 55, learned that he has Parkinson's disease. He had had a tremor for many months, and when it grew more persistent and became accompanied by stiffness and other discomfort,

---

*Concierge medicine is also known by the terms "boutique medicine," "retainer-based medicine," or "direct care medicine."

Andy decided it was time to see a neurologist. We had been anxious for days before the appointment. Hours of Internet searches encouraged us to cling to the hope that the tremor was benign, as many are. But we also knew that we could get life-changing news from the doctor.

The neurologist did a very thorough examination. Then, without indicating that he was ready to deliver his decree, he blurted out, "Well, this is clearly Parkinson's disease." He explained that it was an incurable, degenerative, neurologic disease caused by loss of dopamine cells in the brain and that it usually progresses over decades. The doctor discussed a variety of drugs and recommended one for Andy to try first, assuring us that "most patients tolerate this one well." He instructed us to make another appointment in three months and left the exam room to see his next patient.

What followed were some of the most difficult days of our marriage. Life had changed in an instant. We were consumed by fear that our future was bleak and uncertain, that our place in the world had permanently shifted, that our sense of ourselves would never be the same. And our next medical appointment was not for three months.

Although our friends were incredibly patient, affectionate, and encouraging, we were left on our own to construct professional support systems. In the turmoil of the days and weeks after the diagnosis, what Andy needed was someone to call frequently to discuss his symptoms, his reaction to the new medication, and his mood. He very much would have appreciated having access to a nurse practitioner or a physician assistant who could spend time providing reassurance that this disease could be managed and that life could go on. Waiting for several months for our next contact with a medical professional was not a viable option.

I don't think Andy's doctor was atypical or that he deviated from standard protocol. But patients receiving life-changing diagnoses need much more intensive attention, and they need to benefit from a team approach. In 1994, when my mother became a breast cancer patient at M.D. Anderson Cancer Center in Houston, a social worker literally ran after us as we left one of the first doctors' appointments to make sure that we learned about a variety of resources that the cancer center offered to promote patients' mental and emotional well-being. How I wish that all medical centers adopted similar practices!

According to experts, up to 60 percent of Parkinson's disease patients experience depression. Overlooking these symptoms can have devastating consequences for them. We took initiative, sought a second opinion regarding the diagnosis, and consulted several mental health professionals. But we had to figure out on our own that all this should be done.

Perhaps the most important part of planning for proper medical care in old age is to learn to become an active participant in your own medical care. Doctors have approximately 15 minutes to spend with each patient during a typical office visit.[38] The patient, therefore, needs to feel empowered to guide the physician and to be a key member of his or her medical team.

This principle applies not only to what happens after a serious diagnosis but also to the doctor's visit itself. When a doctor prescribes a medication or recommends a treatment course, the patient should ask questions. How will this drug interact with others that I'm taking? I'm already on several other daily medications, is it really necessary to add another? You are recommending aggressive intervention (e.g., surgery), but are there other options that I should consider first? When accompanying relatives to medical appointments, I have found the following cliché but pointed question to be particularly effective: If this were your mother or sister, which alternative would you select for her?

In the book *When Doctors Don't Listen*, Leana Wen and Joshua Kosowsky develop a set of recommendations to help patients avoid misdiagnosis and unnecessary tests. Their "8 Pillars to Better Diagnosis" are:

1. Tell your whole story;
2. Assert yourself in the doctor's thought process;
3. Participate in your physical exam;
4. Make the differential diagnosis together;
5. Partner for the decision-making process;
6. Apply tests rationally;
7. Use common sense to confirm the working diagnosis;
8. Integrate diagnosis into the healing process.[39]

Central to their book is the assertion that the patient must transform "from being a passive participant who answers yes or no, and submits to tests to being an active storyteller and equal partner in the diagnostic process."[40]

Other commentators refer to an approach of "shared decision making." They urge clinicians to employ decision aids in written, audiovisual, or web-based form to educate patients and families about treatment options, outcomes, risks, and costs.[41] Such educational efforts may improve care, better align treatment with patient preferences, and even reduce costs. Studies have shown that patients participating in shared decision making more frequently select less aggressive, more conservative care options, though it is not clear that these choices consistently lead to better outcomes.[42]

Patients' reluctance to ask their doctors questions has been labeled "white coat silence," and experts have blamed both patients and physicians for this phenomenon. In response, the Agency for Healthcare Research and Quality launched the "Questions Are the Answer" initiative in September 2011. Through marketing outreach it hopes to promote patient engagement and improved communication in the clinical setting.[43]

The Internet is also an invaluable resource for medical information. Baby boomers are largely comfortable with navigating the Internet, and there is nothing wrong with conducting background research before going to the doctor. Although not all websites are reliable, many are managed by very reputable entities, such as the National Institutes of Health, the Centers for Disease Control and Prevention, the American Medical Association, and various prestigious professional organizations. When my mother suffered from her mysterious and precipitous mental deterioration, we learned a great deal about possible causes and remedies through simple Google searches. Years earlier, I was able to self-diagnose a thyroid problem based on several common symptoms. I made an appointment with my internist and asked him to test for a thyroid disorder before trying to explore other possibilities.

Of course, Internet searches should not replace consultation with medical experts, and you should recognize their pitfalls. You should not panic based on what you have learned from the Internet and torment yourself with thoughts of disability and death before you have even been examined by a physician. You should not go to the doctor with a closed mind, convinced that you know exactly what your malady is and what treatment you require. However, research can equip patients to discuss their symptoms more intelligently, ask the right questions, and have more productive and satisfying visits with their health care providers.

If you receive a serious diagnosis, reading relevant literature and communicating with similar patients through Facebook, blogs, support groups, or other means can be invaluable. Ask your doctor to recommend reliable websites, books, support groups, and additional resources. The best advice, however, often comes from fellow patients who have coped with the illness and navigated through treatment longer than you have, and thus, finding ways to connect with them is well worth the effort.

Involving Trusted Advocates and Obtaining Adequate Support

Patients who are too ill or mentally impaired to participate fully in their own medical decision making will need to have an advocate. As indicated in Chapter 4, this arrangement should be formalized through a power of attorney document that will authorize a proxy to make medical decisions if the principal becomes incompetent.

However, regardless of mental status, at least one close friend or relative should be involved whenever a patient of any age is having surgery or suffering from a serious illness. If no friend or relative is available, a geriatric care manager can be employed to be the patient's advocate and care coordinator.[44]

My rules of thumb for my own medical care and that of family members are: (1) don't be shy about sharing health problems with loved ones and asking for reasonable assistance, and (2) don't go to any important medical appointment or to the hospital alone. It is important to have another individual in the room to hear the doctors' explanations, take notes, formulate appropriate questions, and help you review what happened during the medical encounter. In the hospital, it is also important to have someone who can find the nurses when they don't respond to the call button quickly, urge nurses to page the doctor in order to ask for further measures to relieve discomfort, and pose appropriate questions about treatment and prognosis whenever a doctor pops in briefly. As I learned from my experience of caring for my mother through breast cancer just five months after she rushed to my side for my surgery, there will be plenty of opportunities in life to reciprocate.

Undergoing major medical procedures can be particularly challenging for individuals without relatives or friends who can meet their care needs. Short-term paid help from home care agencies is often the answer in such circumstances. Although the cost of $19 per hour[45] may be unaffordable in the long run, having an attentive aide when one is incapacitated for a few days may well be worth the investment. On average, home care agencies require that their aides be hired for a minimum of four hours, though some have no hourly minimum.[46] Service can usually be requested on short notice. Aides can be employed to accompany clients to out-patient procedures, to stay with recuperating patients at home for a few days after surgery, or even to sit in the hospital room with a patient whose discomfort, anxiety, or other needs are unlikely to be fully addressed by the nursing staff on a busy hospital floor. The option of acquiring temporary paid help through an agency is one that I keep on my radar screen for myself and that I find particularly reassuring.

Those who learn to be active members of their own care team earlier in life will be well served as they age. Forming the habits of doing background research, asking educated questions, involving trusted advocates, obtaining adequate support through paid help, and being assertive when one has clear and reasonable care preferences are important components of planning for old age.

COORDINATED CARE PREPAREDNESS CHECKLIST

- Find an internist whom you trust and with whom you are comfortable, and get regular checkups starting in middle age.
- If you are caring for elderly relatives with complex medical problems, consult a geriatrician if one is available in their area.
- If you are not satisfied with the care you or a loved one is receiving, consider a concierge doctor if this is an affordable option for you.
- Learn to be an active member of your own medical team.
  - Before visiting the doctor, do your research (but don't panic about anything you read on the Internet).

- ○ Prepare questions before your appointment, and during your visit with the doctor, don't be afraid to ask questions regarding your symptoms, diagnosis, and the prescribed treatment.
- ○ If you receive a serious diagnosis, seek a second opinion and consult mental health professionals even if this is not suggested by your doctor.
- When you have acute medical problems, obtain adequate support. Have someone accompany you to medical appointments and to the hospital. Hire help during your recovery period if family members or friends are unavailable and you can afford to do so.

7

Long-Term Care

As much as we all hope to avoid it, many of us will need professional long-term care at some point in our lives. Those of us with aging parents are likely to face a decision about obtaining long-term care for them in the last years of their lives, and we may well need the same for ourselves in the future.

Experts expect that as many as seven out of 10 people who are currently 65 or older will eventually require this type of care. Expenditures on such care in the United States totaled $240 billion in 2009, accounting for almost 9 percent of total health care spending.[1] During that year, an estimated 8 million elderly people received paid long-term care services, averaging $30,000 per person, and the number of recipients is expected to rise to 10 million by 2020.[2]

A minority of elderly people have most or all of their care needs met by relatives. It is estimated that almost a quarter of current retirees will receive informal care from family members in their homes for at least two years. In 2006, 30 to 38 million informal caregivers provided care valued at $354 billion.[3]

But even those with strong support systems and dedicated, knowledgeable informal caregivers can face significant challenges as their frailties and needs become more acute. Beth Ann Swan, a nursing school dean, described the obstacles she and her husband faced after his stroke in a 2012 article published in *Health Affairs*.[4] "How can we expect not-yet-well people to suddenly begin managing all of the complex medical and personal issues that just the day before were being handled by an entire team of trained professionals?" she asks as she describes her husband's transition from a rehabilitation hospital to home. For those with no family members to help, the situation can be all the more difficult.

What options are available to older adults who can no longer manage to live independently with or without help from unpaid caregivers such as spouses or children? The choices come down to nursing homes, assisted living, and paid home care obtained through agencies or by independently hiring caregivers.

NURSING HOMES

Sadly, many of my visits with elderly relatives in nursing homes have been discouraging. The few facilities I have seen over the years seemed understaffed, and the residents complained that they did not receive prompt attention when they needed to use the bathroom, to obtain medication for pain relief, or to be transported to another area of the nursing home. In one case, patients with dementia were strapped to wheelchairs and placed around the nursing station so that nurses did not have to walk to different rooms to check on them. My relatives complained that showers were allowed only twice a week and must be taken in the middle of the night because night shift staff members are less busy than day shift personnel. To the extent that activities were offered, many were not intellectually stimulating and seemed more appropriate for small children than adults. Residents who had their full mental faculties had few opportunities for social interaction because so many of the other residents had some degree of dementia or were otherwise unable or unwilling to form new friendships.

My mother-in-law, Helen, complained bitterly about the lack of social opportunities during a two-month stay in a nursing home in which she received physical therapy after a fall. One day, after learning how to maneuver on her own in a wheelchair, Helen wheeled herself into a common room and was glad to see a fellow patient sitting on a sofa. The woman motioned to Helen to come close and then grabbed Helen's hand and put it to her own face, clearly craving another human being's touch. When Helen asked for the woman's name, she was able to say "Mary" but was not able to converse any further. Helen saw Mary the next day and said hello, but the woman stared at her blankly without any recognition.

Yet nursing home stays are sometimes a necessary and welcome step to recovery from a medical crisis. Nursing homes provide skilled nursing services, that is, care by licensed practitioners who are available 24 hours a day. A large percentage of us will have at least a short sojourn in a nursing home. Experts estimate that between 35 and 50 percent of those who are 65 or older will reside in nursing homes at some point in their lives. Patients often use nursing homes temporarily while recovering from a debilitating illness, injury, or surgery in order to receive wound care, physical and occupational therapy, or tube feeding.[5]

Others move to a nursing home at the end of life because it is the only safe option for them. Permanent nursing home residents are among the most frail elderly. Most commonly, they are there because they have severe dementia, incontinence, behavioral problems, or no family.[6]

Typically, even permanent residents do not live very long in nursing homes. A 2010 study of 1,817 adults who died in nursing homes between 1992 and 2006 revealed that the residents lived in nursing homes for an average of 13.7 months, but 53 percent died within six months of entering the nursing home. Median length of stay varied significantly by gender (men stayed for three months and women for eight months) and net worth (the highest 25 percent stayed for three months and lowest 25 percent for nine months).[7] Only 10 to 20 percent live in nursing homes for more than five years.[8] The relatively short duration of permanent nursing home stays might be attributable to the fact that they are a choice of last resort for many people who move there only when their health has badly deteriorated. Skeptics might also posit that a permanent move to a nursing home does damage to one's will to live, which can hasten death. As Paula Span writes in her book *When the Time Comes*, "[n]obody wants to go to a nursing home, indispensable as they sometimes are; seniors and their families tend to shudder at the very phrase."[9]

Quality of Care

Unfortunately, research confirms that the quality of many nursing homes leaves much to be desired. According to the Kaiser Family Foundation,* on average, U.S. nursing homes had 8.4 deficiencies in 2011.[10] Deficiencies are problems that "can result in a negative impact on the health and safety of residents." The 10 most common deficiencies were categorized as (1) poor infection control (found in 42.7 percent of certified nursing facilities); (2) accident hazards (found in 40.7 percent); (3) inadequate food sanitation (in 36.2 percent); (4) poor quality of care (in 32.5 percent); (5) inadequate individualized comprehensive care plans (in 25.4 percent); (6) unnecessary drugs (in 21.9 percent); (7) failure to meet professional standards (in 20.7 percent); (8) failure to maintain satisfactory clinical records (in 20.3 percent); (9) problems with labeling and storage of drugs, including controlled substances (in 19.5 percent); and (10) failure to promote residents' dignity (in 18.7 percent).[11]

---

*Kaiser analyzed data from the federal On-Line Survey and Certification System (OSCAR) reports that are completed by state licensing and certification programs for the U.S. Centers for Medicare and Medicaid Services.

In 2014, the Department of Health and Human Services Office of Inspector General (OIG) released a startling report that revealed the following:

- Approximately 22 percent of Medicare beneficiaries experienced adverse events during their skilled nursing facility (SNF) stays. An adverse event is defined as one that results in a "prolonged SNF stay or transfer to hospital, permanent harm, life-sustaining intervention, or death."
- An additional 11 percent of Medicare beneficiaries suffered temporary harm while at an SNF. Temporary harm requires intervention but does not cause lasting injury. Examples are light allergic reactions to medications, some falls, and pressure ulcers.
- Fifty-nine percent of incidents were clearly or likely preventable.
- The preventable harm is attributed to "substandard treatment, inadequate resident monitoring, and failure or delay of necessary care."
- Over 50 percent of residents who experienced harm returned to hospitals for treatment, costing Medicare $208 million in August 2011, or an estimated $2.8 billion during fiscal year 2011.[12]

Experts often blame nursing home quality problems on a scarcity of well-trained staff members. Nursing home employees report a disturbing degree of job dissatisfaction, which leads to high turnover rates. In a 2006 survey of over 100,000 such workers, only half stated that they were satisfied with their employment situation. Regulators estimate that acceptable nursing home care requires a minimum of 4.1 hours of nursing time per resident per day, but fewer than 10 percent of nursing homes can meet that standard.[13]

Those without families are the worst off in nursing homes. Family members provide both emotional support and crucial medical and other information to nursing home staff, especially when the patient is cognitively impaired. They also serve an oversight role, ensuring that the patient's needs are met to the extent possible. Staff members in fact are likely to prioritize care for those who receive frequent visits in order to ensure that these patients will appear clean, dressed, and in good spirits to whomever stops by.[14] Therefore, it is important to visit loved ones in nursing homes as frequently as possible and to ask people to visit you if you become a nursing home resident.

According to the Kaiser Family Foundation, in 2010, there were 1.4 million people living in U.S. nursing homes.[15] There were 1.7 million beds in 15,622 certified nursing facilities throughout the United States with an average occupancy rate of 83.3 percent. Among nursing homes, 68 percent were for-profit, 26 percent were nonprofit, and 6 percent were government-owned facilities.

If you or a loved one needs nursing home care, you do not have to leave the quality of the facility up to chance. Rather, you should research nursing homes as thoroughly as possible. A useful resource is "Nursing Home

Compare" on the Medicare.gov website, which features nursing home ratings.[16] Further information can be obtained from the website of your state's health department or by calling the department and requesting any reports it has produced concerning nursing homes that interest you.[17] You should be mindful, however, that federal and state ratings and reports may not be based on comprehensive information. For example, government authorities may rely excessively on self-reporting by nursing homes, fail to take into account significant information such as lawsuits filed by aggrieved patients' family members, and be duped by manipulative practices such as hiring additional staff members right before scheduled inspections and then laying them off.[18] Thus, recommendations from friends who have personal knowledge about nursing homes are particularly valuable, and, if time permits, you should visit potential nursing homes in order to form a firsthand impression of their atmosphere and quality of care. One factor to consider is that there is evidence that nonprofit facilities provide better care than for-profit entities, which may be tempted to cut corners in order to increase their profits.[19]

Costs

One reason for a move to a nursing home is that it may be the only affordable alternative for the very frail because Medicare and Medicaid can cover costs. A 2011 study revealed that on average, a private room in a U.S. nursing home costs $85,775 per year, while patients pay $75,555 annually for a semiprivate nursing home room.[20] However, Medicare covers some of the costs for rehabilitation in a nursing home in limited circumstances.[21] Patients who meet Medicare requirements can receive 20 days of free care per benefit period and then pay a daily copay for days 21 to 100 (up to $152 per day in 2014), after which no Medicare funds are available until the next benefit period.*

To be eligible for Medicare coverage, patients must transfer to a nursing home after having spent at least three consecutive days as admitted patients in a hospital. Some patients remain in the hospital "under observation," and this status does not qualify them for nursing home payment.[22] I learned the meaning of this distinction through my mother-in-law's difficult experience.

---

*Medicare explains the term "benefit period" as follows:

A benefit period begins the day you're admitted as an inpatient in a hospital or [a skilled nursing facility (SNF)]. The benefit period ends when you haven't received any inpatient hospital care (or skilled care in a SNF) for 60 days in a row. If you go into a hospital or a SNF after one benefit period has ended, a new benefit period begins. . . . There's no limit to the number of benefit periods.

"Glossary-B," Medicare.gov, accessed October 21, 2014, http://www.medicare.gov /glossary/b.html.

Observational Status

At the age of 93, my mother-in-law, who lived alone, fell and broke her ankle in three places. We knew that after her hospitalization, she would need to be in a rehabilitation facility until, hopefully, she regained mobility. But on her first full day in the hospital, we received terrible news: my mother-in-law, who was too frail for surgery, was under observation rather than admitted, and thus was considered to be an outpatient. Consequently, she would be ineligible for Medicare coverage of her rehabilitation care and, even during her hospitalization, would incur copayments for doctors' fees and hospital services. She would also have to pay for the many drugs she ordinarily took at home that were now being provided by the hospital.

In some sense, we were lucky to find out that she was only under observation, because hospitals are under no obligation to inform patients of this consequential fact.* After much begging and pleading, the hospital admitted her, much to our relief. Our take-away lesson was that you should always ask whether you are an admitted patient or under observation, and that if you want to change your status to admitted, you should argue with hospital administrators while you are still in the hospital. Going through a Medicare appeal process after the fact is much more time-consuming, burdensome, and frustrating.

Recently, the Centers for Medicare and Medicaid Services issued its "two-midnight rule," which will be enforced starting March 31, 2015. The rule establishes that doctors should admit patients if they expect their stays to last through two midnights, but to list those expected to stay for less time as being under observation. Many have criticized this rule as arbitrary because it will advantage individuals who arrive shortly before midnight (they are more likely to stay a second midnight) and disadvantage those who arrive shortly after midnight, but the rule at least provides some clarity.[23]

Medicaid Eligibility

Although short stays in a nursing home can be covered by Medicare, another public form of insurance, Medicaid, pays for many permanent residencies. Unfortunately, to be eligible for Medicaid coverage, you must "spend down" your assets,[24] and "spending down" is a fairly literal term. It requires you to drain most assets other than your home, personal effects, and vehicle. Detailed guidelines determine Medicaid eligibility, but typically, single people must have no more than $2,000 in "countable resources" (cash, financial accounts, stocks, bonds, and available assets in trust).[25]

---

*This is true in all states but New York, where legislation requires hospitals to inform Medicare beneficiaries of their observation status and allow them to appeal it.

Moreover, individuals cannot simply transfer their assets in order to become Medicaid eligible. The law restricts transfers made during the five years before you apply for Medicaid, a window of time commonly known as the "look-back" period. The law does not prohibit all transfers, but rather, it addresses those made for less than fair market value. For example, if you own jewelry appraised at $30,000, you cannot give it away or sell it for anything less than that amount during the look-back period. Thus, sale of the jewelry should yield $30,000 that you count as assets for Medicaid eligibility purposes.

Transferring assets for less than fair market value during the look-back period does not disqualify you from Medicaid eligibility forever, but it will result in a penalty period. To calculate the length of this period, divide the overall value of the assets you transferred or undersold by the average monthly cost of a nursing home in your state. For example, if you gave away $30,000 in assets, and the average cost of a nursing home in your state is $6,000 per month, you would be ineligible for Medicaid for five months ($30,000 divided by $6,000). The penalty period usually begins on the date of application for Medicaid, assuming you meet all other requirements.[26]

Be aware that spouses who have considerable separate assets will not be able to retain all of those assets if their sick spouse wishes to enroll in Medicaid for purposes of nursing home care. When a married couple applies for Medicaid, a snapshot is taken of the couple's total assets, whether they are held jointly or separately. Medicaid disregards prenuptial agreements. State law will allow the "community spouse" (the healthy person who continues to live in the community) to keep a "community spouse resource allowance." In 2014, this amount ranged from a maximum of $117,240 to a minimum of $23,448 depending on the state. State law also addresses the amount of income working community spouses may keep from their ongoing earnings or, if they have little to no monthly income, the amount they may obtain from their institutionalized spouses' incomes to meet their living expenses. These amounts may vary significantly from state to state.[27]

In 2010, 63 percent of nursing home residents were covered by Medicaid, 14 percent were covered by Medicare, and 22 percent paid from private sources.[28] Sadly, according to one study, individuals who have lived in a nursing home for six months or more were found to have a median total household wealth of only $5,518.[29] Thus, many people who have worked hard for their earnings and take pride in having money to leave as an inheritance for their loved ones must instead hand over their life savings to nursing home operators.

ASSISTED LIVING

Seniors who are in decline but do not need skilled nursing care may opt for assisted living settings. These facilities allow residents to have their own apartments or rooms along with assistance that is available around the clock, including prepared meals, cleaning services, activities, transportation, and some health care.[30] They do not, however, provide skilled nursing services.

Assisted living offers seniors a more active, autonomous life than nursing homes. Residents often have apartments rather than rooms and can cook for themselves if they wish. Nevertheless, seniors are rarely enthusiastic about leaving their homes for an assisted living facility and most often do not enter assisted living settings until they are simply unable to live on their own. More than half of the 733,300 people in assisted living in 2010 were 85 and older.[31] Almost 40 percent of residents received assistance with three or more activities of daily living, over 40 percent had Alzheimer's disease or other dementias, and perhaps as many as 90 percent had at least mild cognitive impairment.[32] Residents reportedly take an average of nine drugs per day, including both prescription and over-the-counter medications.[33]

The cost of assisted living is a significant barrier for many consumers. In 2013, the average total monthly charge per resident for assisted living care in the United States was approximately $3,500.[34] Prices can vary greatly by region. For example, in 2008, the monthly price tag was approximately $2,200 in South Dakota and over $4,500 in Chicago.[35] Facilities may also charge additional fees for extra services. Assisted living is generally paid for out of pocket, and Medicaid provides some degree of coverage for only 19 percent of residents.[36] Consequently, assisted living residents who exhaust their financial resources may be transferred to nursing homes for which Medicaid will pay.

The residents' median length of stay was 671 days in 2010, that is, approximately 22 months.[37] About a third of residents die in assisted living, but a larger percentage transfer to nursing homes as their health fails (or finances dwindle). Residents may in fact be involuntarily discharged from assisted living as their needs intensify.[38] Because seniors often do not move to assisted living until their eighties, when they are physically or mentally frail, these facilities may not provide a robust social setting and frequently constitute a temporary rather than a permanent, final home. In the words of the writer Paula Span, assisted living is sometimes "sardonically called a nursing home with a chandelier."[39]

Although patients may enter nursing homes directly from the hospital, leaving very little time for extensive investigation of choices, the same is not true for assisted living facilities. The decision to move to assisted living is generally made without the pressure of an emergency or acute medical needs so that you should have adequate time to explore alternatives. Websites such as Angie's List and Caring.com provide reviews and ratings. States often survey assisted living facilities as part of their regulatory enforcement process and some post surveys on their websites. In addition, you may call your state's department of health and request any assessments it has concerning facilities in which you are interested.[40] You should also seek recommendations from friends and acquaintances and visit assisted living centers that you are considering.

HOME CARE AGENCIES

About 96 percent of adults who are 65 and older live in noninstitutional settings, and the vast majority wish to live out their lives in their own homes.[41] Even among those 85 and older, fewer than 20 percent enter nursing homes.[42] A popular option for such individuals is home care.

Home care is supportive care that is provided to the elderly in their own homes. The terminology for this type of care, however, can be confusing and is inconsistently used. Some states differentiate between "home health care," which includes visits by licensed medical personnel such as those providing skilled nursing or rehabilitation services, and "in-home care," which covers a lower level of services. In-home care may include companionship, assistance with daily living activities (e.g., cooking, dressing, and bathing), driving, and medication reminders.[43]

In 2012, Americans spent an estimated $77.8 billion on home care.[44] In 2010, there were over 10,800 Medicare-certified home health agencies benefiting 3.4 million patients who receive over 122.5 million home care visits.[45] In 2013, the average cost of home health care in the United States was $19 per hour.[46]

Medicare pays for limited home care for homebound elderly people. Services may include skilled nursing, physical therapy, social services, and assistance with activities of daily living for up to 28 hours a week for a limited period of time, typically after discharge from a hospital or rehabilitation facility.[47] In some states, Medicaid also provides some degree of home care coverage for Medicaid-eligible low income patients,[48] and support may also be available through local programs, charities, or the Veterans' Administration.

An aide hired through a home care agency can be a very good solution for frail elderly people who live alone and wish to avoid moving to an institutional setting. Agencies ideally screen employees, supervise workers, dispatch substitutes if assigned aides become unavailable, and allow clients to request personnel changes when they are dissatisfied with particular aides. Agencies also handle all of the paperwork, which can be an invaluable service to elderly individuals who are trying to navigate the system on their own.

Nevertheless, while agency-provided home care allows the elderly to remain in their homes, this approach too has its drawbacks. The cost is an obvious barrier, but it is not the only concern. Home care aides are largely female, minority, and immigrant, and they are often underpaid and overworked. Their average hourly wage in 2012 was $10.50, and the average annual salary was $21,750.[49] Consequently, their annual turnover rate is considerable, perhaps as high as 60 percent. Having to get used to new caregivers on a frequent basis can be distressing, especially for people with dementia. In addition, agencies might have somewhat rigid policies, such as refusing to allow workers to drive clients for fear of liability or requiring that aides be used for a minimum number of weekly hours.

Regulatory oversight and compliance are yet another concern. Medicare oversees home health care agencies that provide skilled nursing care, physical therapy, occupational therapy, speech therapy, medical social services, and home health aide services. The Medicare website provides useful quality surveys on certified home health agencies.* However, agencies that provide less skilled services are not governed by Medicare rules. Some states post similar information about in-home care agencies on their websites, but others do not regulate in-home care agencies at all. Furthermore, even states with robust regulations often have inadequate enforcement resources, and, therefore, they cannot effectively prevent or punish most violations of the law.

Before employing aides from a home care agency, you should do as much research as possible. This includes not only looking for rankings and quality surveys on the Internet, but also asking acquaintances for recommendations based on personal experience. Ascertaining the quality of the agency is especially important if your loved one is mentally impaired and will not be able to explain his or her needs to the caregiver, advocate for him- or herself, or report that he or she is dissatisfied with the care being given. In-home care aides spend many hours alone with their clients and have their clients' welfare and, frequently, even lives in their hands. Thus, the decision to employ a particular agency cannot be taken lightly.

Hiring Aides Independently

A less expensive and more flexible alternative to using an agency is to hire an aide independently. According to Paula Span, "[m]ore people hire home care independently (through what's been called the gray market) than through agencies."[50] Independent hiring can be initiated by posting an ad through Internet services such as Craigslist or Care.com. Some states, such as Oregon, also have state-run registries that enable workers and employers to specify their criteria and conduct searches in order to be matched.[51]

However, this may be an overwhelming undertaking for many seniors and impossible for those with cognitive impairment and no family support. A sound hiring process entails advertising, interviewing, performing background and reference checks, and formulating a detailed contract. Because

---

*They are available at http://www.medicare.gov/HomeHealthCompare/search.aspx.

individuals who respond to ads on Craigslist or Care.com are not licensed or screened, conducting reference calls and a background check through a reliable service is essential. Once a caregiver is selected, the contract should specify tasks, hours, payment, conditions for termination, and the terms of a short probationary or trial period during which the client can determine whether satisfactory services are being provided.[52] In addition, those who employ aides independently will need to arrange to pay social security and state unemployment compensation taxes.

After my mother died, my 86-year-old father, who suffered from congestive heart failure, decided that he wanted to stay in his home but was not prepared to live alone. He wanted to hire a male caregiver who would sleep at the house, provide transportation, help with household chores, and serve as a companion.

We initially met with a home health care agency and learned that round-the-clock service would cost up to $480 per day or approximately $175,000 per year. In order to find a less expensive alternative, we posted an ad on Craigslist. A young man in his mid-20s responded with an articulate and compelling e-mail explaining why he was interested in the job. We interviewed him twice, conducted a criminal background check through the Internet, called his references, and hired him for $20,000 a year plus room and board.

Although calling references is helpful, other research, including a Google search and a thorough background check, is critical. Remember, the applicant is providing the names of references, and, therefore, you can assume that the individuals you call think highly of him or her. Nevertheless, you should make the phone calls because you may be able to evaluate the references' level of enthusiasm about the candidate from their tone or wording. To further judge their credibility, you may want to ask surprising questions, such as "Please tell me two negative things about the applicant."

A simple Google search of the candidate's name may reveal very useful information, such as whether the person has been involved in litigation and what prior jobs he or she has had. Searching Facebook and other social media can be equally productive. For the background check we used a service called Intelius, which produces a report based on the last name and the person's social security number for $49.95.* The website advertises that its reports include, when available, "statewide criminal check, address history, relatives and roommates, neighbors, home value and details, neighborhood info, satellite and map images, alias names," and more.

At the time, my father did not have severe cognitive impairment, and one of my sisters lived 10 minutes away and could visit him almost daily,

---

*It is available at https://www.intelius.com/purchase.php.

so the risk of elder abuse or neglect seemed small. Happily, my father was pleased with his live-in caregiver for over a year. This came as a shock to many acquaintances who had warned me that it was nearly impossible to find a good aide on the first try and that their relatives had fired one individual after another, usually after trial periods that lasted just days. When my father's health deteriorated and he began to require constant attention, we switched to round-the-clock care supplied by a home care agency.

A potential concern stemming from all forms of home care is that it will cause the elderly person to become socially isolated. If the individual does not receive regular visits from friends and family members, the aide may be the only one with whom the client interacts in person for weeks at a time. Experts who have studied the benefits of social contact have found that interaction with hired personnel is not as beneficial as naturally occurring social relationships.[53] Caregivers should thus be asked to help clients remain active in religious or other community organizations or become newly involved in appropriate activities, such as those offered by senior centers. According to the National Council on Aging, almost 11,000 senior centers exist in the United States and serve 1 million individuals every day.[54]

As in every other setting, quality of care is of serious concern. Both agencies and independently employed aides can provide subpar services. In extreme cases, they may even engage in elder abuse. According to the National Center on Elder Abuse, there are no accurate figures as to how many elderly people are abused or neglected because only a small fraction of cases are reported. Some studies estimate that 7.6 to 10 percent of the elderly are victims, though this figure does not include financial exploitation, and in as many as 90 percent of cases, the abuser is a relative.[55] Seniors with cognitive impairment and those without frequent visitors may be particularly vulnerable to receiving less-than-optimal services from a caregiver. Unannounced visits by friends and family members are an invaluable form of oversight and quality control.

PART-TIME CARE: ADULT DAY SERVICES

Those seeking part-time care for their loved ones should consider one additional option—adult day services. Over 5,000 adult day service facilities exist, benefiting 260,000 seniors and their caregivers.[56] There are two types of adult day care: adult social day care, which emphasizes social activities, meals, and recreation, and adult day health care, which offers more intensive therapeutic and social services for individuals who suffer from serious problems such as diabetes, hypertension, stroke, and dementia.

Adult day health care may be used for short-term, posthospitalization care and rehabilitation or as a longer-term solution for frail elderly people. For the latter group, it can supplement or replace in-home care and also delay or avoid placement in assisted living or skilled nursing facilities. Both types of adult day services provide participants with a large number of services and allow family caregivers to retain their own jobs or enjoy free time while their loved one receives care in a safe setting.

Adult day service centers offer health monitoring, social opportunities, activities, and assistance with daily functions. Approximately 80 percent have a nurse on staff; about half have a social worker; half also offer physical, occupational, or speech therapy; and 60 percent provide case management services. The majority have special programs for dementia patients. They also offer caregiver support in the form of education, support groups, and counseling. According to a national study, the care worker-to-participant ratio is one to six, which promotes significant personal attention.[57]

Adult day services charge an average of $71 per day.[58] Many clients must pay out of pocket, but in some cases, public programs such as Medicaid, the Veterans' Administration, or state social services will pay part or all of the expense, depending on the client's income and eligibility. Private medical insurance policies might also cover a portion of adult day care center costs if licensed medical professionals provide care, and long-term care insurance policies often provide coverage as well.[59]

The National Adult Day Services Association urges seniors and their caregivers to visit facilities (perhaps more than once) and speak to participants before making their selection. The association also recommends that you ask the following questions:

- How many years has the center been in operation?
- Does the center have a license, certification, or accreditation?
- What are the hours of operation?
- Are transportation services offered?
- What is the cost?
- Is it an hourly or daily charge? Are there other charges?
- What types of payment are accepted?
- Is financial assistance available?
- Is specialized care provided for conditions such as memory loss?
- What is the staff-to-client ratio?
- What kinds of training do staff receive?
- Do participants have access to services such as physical or occupational therapy?
- What types of activities are provided?
- Are meals or snacks provided? Are special diets accommodated?[60]

Although some states regulate adult day service centers and require licenses and certification, others do not. You can find local adult day service centers through online resources such as Helpguide.org* or your state's adult day services association.[61] You may also contact your local Area Agency on Aging for a list of nearby facilities.†

LONG-TERM CARE PREPAREDNESS CHECKLIST

- If you or a loved one will require rehabilitation care after a hospitalization, inquire as to whether the patient is admitted or under observation prior to leaving the hospital. Be aware that Medicare will not pay for inpatient rehabilitation unless the patient was admitted and stayed in the hospital for at least three days.
- Do your research before selecting a nursing home, assisted living facility, home care agency, or adult day services centers. Search the Internet, seek word-of-mouth recommendations, and visit the facilities in person.
- If you want to avoid institutionalization, consider obtaining home care either through an agency or by hiring a caregiver independently.
- Consider supplementing care by family members or paid aides with care at adult day services.
- If you hire a caregiver on your own, be sure to call references, Google the applicant, and conduct a comprehensive background check using a reputable Internet service.
- Visit loved ones who are receiving care in nursing homes, assisted living, or at home as frequently as possible. Ask friends and family members to visit you if you are the one needing care.

---

*At htttp://www.helpguide.org/elder/adult_day_care_centers.htm.
†Information can be obtained by calling 800-677-1116.

8

Exit Strategies: Maintaining Control at the End of Life

Most of this book has focused on planning for living a fulfilling and comfortable life in old age. Old age, however, inevitably ends in death. What, if any, planning can or should be done for the end of life's journey?

Few individuals die suddenly without some period of physical or cognitive decline. According to one study of nearly 8,000 deaths among Medicare beneficiaries, only 7 percent died "suddenly," which was defined as "progressing from normal functioning to death in a brief time . . . [with] little forewarning and often little or no interaction with the healthcare system before dying."[1] A second study involved 4,190 individuals who were interviewed during their last year of life or whose decision-making agents were interviewed. The researchers concluded that 15 percent of the subjects experienced sudden death, meaning that they had no diagnosis of cancer, heart disease, diabetes, hip fracture, or stroke when they died and no nursing home stay.[2]

Although longevity is generally perceived as a blessing, many who have watched the decline of elderly loved ones are more dubious about its benefits. A prolonged existence devoid of the ability to enjoy even simple pleasures can hardly be described as good fortune. The hero of Jonathan Swift's *Gulliver's Travels* describes the "Stulbrugs" or "Immortals" about which he learned during one of his voyages:

At Ninety they lose their Teeth and Hair; they have at that Age no Distinction of Taste, but eat and drink whatever they can get, without Relish or Appetite. The Diseases they were subject to, still continue without increasing or diminishing. In talking they forget the common Appellation of Things, and the Names of Persons, even of those who are their nearest Friends and Relations. For the same Reason they never can amuse themselves with reading, because their Memory will not serve to carry them from the Beginning of a Sentence to the End; and by this Defect they are deprived of the only Entertainment whereof they might otherwise be capable.[3]

This description is fictional, but for one of my relatives, Mae, who lived to be 104, it was quite apt during the last 18 months of her life. Mae and her sister Nettie, who was five years younger, lived in different apartments in the same building in Cleveland, each with round-the-clock aides hired through a home care agency. They visited each other daily, enjoyed occasional outings, and sometimes talked about how Nettie would move to Boston after Mae's death so she could be closer to her son and grandchildren. Nettie, however, died in 2011 at age 96 from breast cancer that was not diagnosed until she had a tumor the size of a large apricot breaking through her skin. Although she visited her internist every few months, she said he spent only a couple of minutes with her, taking her blood pressure and listening to her heart. Because the doctor never asked if anything else was wrong, Nettie thought it was inappropriate to trouble him with a question about the growing lump in her breast.

At 102, Mae, who had never married, was inconsolable. She spent large portions of the day sleeping, lost her appetite, and exhibited rapid mental deterioration. During her last few months, it was unclear whether she recognized her visitors, and she did not remember even the simple details of her life, such as where she lived and what relatives she had. On good days, she could ask a question such as "How are your parents?" but she asked it repeatedly throughout the visit. She also expressed her profound distress about her circumstances, uttering phrases such as, "I never thought this would happen to me," "I wouldn't wish this on my worst enemy," and "My whole family is gone." Mae died on her 104th birthday because of fluid on her lungs.

Mae was never combative or uncooperative with caregivers. However, I have seen first-hand that other dementia patients can become hostile, verbally abusive, and even violent with paid caregivers and loved ones alike. For family members, it can be agonizing to watch relatives who were gentle souls and highly respected professionals undergo a radical change in personality at the end of life.

Some acquaintances have told me that they or their relatives have a concrete plan to commit suicide at a particular age (e.g., 85) or at the first sign of dementia. This approach has even been discussed in academic literature. For example, Professor Dena Davis, a bioethics scholar who teaches at Lehigh University, has argued that "suicide is one rational response to the knowledge that one will have Huntington's disease or Alzheimer's disease."[4] It is noteworthy that in 2010, approximately 18 percent of suicides were reportedly committed by individuals who were 85 or older.[5]

In contrast, other individuals are certain that every moment of life is precious and emphasize the sanctity of human life. They would not consider any acts to shorten their lives because they view such acts as morally impermissible.[6] Perhaps they are in an enviable position because they are free of moral uncertainty and the need to make difficult end-of-life decisions.

Still others, myself included, occupy a middle ground. Formulating a plan to commit suicide before suffering significant age-related deterioration is out of the question for any number of reasons: religion, culture, social norms, lack of courage. Yet, we contemplate with horror the prospect of having no control over our fate at the end of life, no matter what suffering befalls us. As a 29-year-old, I developed a very large, borderline malignant ovarian tumor, as described in the introduction to this book. Before surgery, I endured nearly unbearable pain and, years later, experienced several episodes of similar pain because of internal scar tissue. If such agony were long lasting and could not be stopped through medical interventions, I could well imagine wanting my life to end and contemplating doing something about it.

So now back to the original question: Can any planning be done to reduce suffering before death? To that end, with what existing options and interventions should middle-aged individuals become familiar and for what further choices might they lobby?

PHYSICIAN-ASSISTED AND NON-PHYSICIAN-ASSISTED SUICIDE BY DYING PATIENTS

The most aggressive means of maintaining control in the last months of life while still benefiting from the involvement of medical professionals is physician-assisted suicide. This is an option in just a handful of states in this country. Oregon, Washington, and Vermont legalized the practice by statute in 1994, 2008, and 2013, respectively.[7] In 2009, Montana's Supreme Court held that physicians who provide aid in dying pursuant to patients' wishes are immune from criminal liability, though the state has not established a legal protocol for the practice.[8] In 2014, a lower court in New Mexico likewise affirmed a patient's right to choose aid in dying.

In truth, very few people end their lives through legal assisted suicide. According to Oregon's Death with Dignity Act's (DWDA) 2013 report:

As of January 22, 2014, prescriptions for lethal medications were written for 122 people during 2013 under the provisions of the DWDA, compared to 116 during 2012. . . . At the time of this report, there were 71 known DWDA deaths during 2013. This corresponds to 21.9 DWDA deaths per 10,000 total deaths.[9]

Washington State reported that in 2013, 173 patients received medication pursuant to its Death with Dignity Act. Of these, 159 died, but only 119 are known to have ingested the medication. The others died of natural or unknown causes. Washington provides these further details concerning the 104 deceased individuals: they ranged in age from 29 to 95; 77 percent had cancer; 15 percent had neurodegenerative disease, including Lou Gehrig's disease; and 8 percent had heart and respiratory disease or other illnesses.[10]

The small number of patients who complete assisted suicide is attributable to several factors. First, a large percentage of residents in the states that have passed physician-assisted suicide are opposed to the practice's legalization. In Oregon, a full 40 percent voted against it in 1997. According to Oregon officials who interviewed a large number of state residents, only 20 percent of individuals who died in 2000–2002 at the ages of 65 to 84 told family members that they personally considered physician-assisted suicide.[11] Like ordinary citizens, physicians themselves may oppose the practice, and if they do, they are free to refuse to write prescriptions for the necessary drugs. Thus, some patients who would be interested in pursuing the option but live in remote areas or small towns may not be able to find a doctor to help them.

Second, the statutes establish strict eligibility criteria for patients seeking physician-assisted suicide. The patient must be at least 18 years old, a resident of the state, able to make and communicate health care decisions him- or herself, and diagnosed by two physicians as having a terminal illness that will lead to death within six months. Experts note that it is often very difficult to predict with any degree of confidence when death will occur.[12] If either the attending or consulting physician determines that the patient's judgment is impaired by depression or another condition, the individual must undergo a psychological examination. It is noteworthy that patients with dementia are ineligible for physician-assisted suicide because the statutes do not permit substitute decision making or allow physicians to honor requests for physician-assisted suicide that were made in advance directives. The attending physician must be licensed in the state; must inform the patient of alternatives such as palliative care; and, in Oregon and Washington, must ask patients to notify their next of kin of their prescription requests.

The request procedures are also somewhat elaborate. There is a mandatory 15-day waiting period between a first and second oral request to a physician followed by submission of a written request to the doctor. In addition, there is a 48-hour waiting period before picking up the prescription from a pharmacy. In Oregon and Washington, physicians must report to the state all prescriptions that they write for assisted suicide purposes.

Finally, the statistics reported by Oregon and Washington* suggest that in about one-third of cases, individuals find comfort in having the option of taking the drugs but die naturally before deciding to actually do so. For some, taking the irreversible step of initiating death may turn out to be more complicated or frightening than they thought it would be.

Residents of states in which physician-assisted suicide is not legal are left to their own devices if they wish to end their lives before they die naturally. A variety of websites and publications offer chemical and drug recipes and equipment that aim to help patients end their lives as painlessly as possible. The Hemlock Society was famous for serving as a resource for aid in dying, but it has merged with another group and is now called Compassion & Choices. One of the services discussed on Compassion & Choices' website is "end-of-life consultation."[13] Experts warn that those following suicide manuals on their own are at risk of making mistakes that can render them seriously disabled but still alive. This is because "underlying disease states and chronic drug therapy may affect the absorption, distribution, metabolism and excretion of substances ingested."[14]

Americans may have one option for physician-assisted suicide outside of the United States. Dignitas is a Swiss organization founded in 1998 that accepts clients from all over the world for purposes of assisted suicide at a facility in Zurich. According to its website, it uses a fast-acting and painless barbiturate dissolved in drinking water. To qualify for "accompanied suicide" an individual must be a member of Dignitas, of sound judgment, able to self-administer the drug, and have one of the following: (1) a terminal illness, (2) "unendurable incapacitating disability," or (3) "unbearable and uncontrollable pain."[15] A film called The Suicide Tourist (available on YouTube) portrays Dignitas in a very positive light. However, not surprisingly, the organization has been controversial and occasionally faces misconduct accusations. Nevertheless, a study published in the Journal of Medical Ethics[16] found that "suicide tourism" to Switzerland had doubled between 2009 and 2012.

In most states in the United States, physicians whose patients seek their aid in dying can do little more than advise them to stop eating and drinking. Death from starvation and dehydration can take seven to 10 days or longer. This seems like a terrible way to die, but there are a number of published accounts of patients who have made this choice. A particularly poignant one is Zoe FitzGerald Carter's Imperfect Endings. In this book, she recounts

---

*Montana and Vermont do not post statistics. New Mexico's assisted suicide decision came from a lower court and was appealed. As of this writing, no appellate decision has been issued in the case.

the story of her mother, a long-time Parkinson's disease sufferer with very advanced disease, who died after 12 days of fasting supplemented by a morphine overdose.[17]

What about patients with dementia who do not have the capacity to decide to stop eating and drinking? One controversial approach is to address the matter in your advance directive. Two scholars, Paul. T. Menzel and M. Colette Chandler-Cramer, have argued that individuals should be able to direct that they not be given food and water if they have severe dementia and resist being fed or show no signs of enjoying the activity of eating. The authors write that "with an appropriate directive, full withholding is [ethically] justified when the current experiential value of survival to the patient has diminished enough that it is outweighed by the critical interests and autonomy represented in the directive."[18] Other ethicists would find this approach morally unacceptable and posit that patients with dementia should be fed as long as eating and drinking does not cause them real distress.[19] If you feel that you would want to have food and water withheld if you develop severe dementia and no longer enjoy eating, you should certainly address the matter in your advance directive. However, my guess would be that many caregivers would feel too uncomfortable to honor this instruction.

PALLIATIVE AND HOSPICE CARE

Hospice is a far less controversial approach than physician-assisted suicide to avoiding unwanted life-prolonging treatment at the end of life. Hospice care is available to terminally ill patients and provides treatment that promotes comfort but is not designed to cure their illnesses. Thus, hospice patients do not undergo aggressive curative therapies such as chemotherapy and radiation and are not taken to the hospital for medical care. They do receive plenty of medications to address pain, nausea, shortness of breath, and other sources of discomfort. To be eligible, patients must obtain certification from their doctors and hospice directors that they have a terminal illness and are expected to die within six months.[20]

Palliative care, also known as comfort care, is available not only to hospice patients but also to those who wish to receive curative therapies at the same time. Palliative care focuses on relieving discomfort caused by pain, shortness of breath, fatigue, insomnia, digestive problems, nausea, loss of appetite, and stress.[21] Palliative care specialists may refer patients to psychologists or even to attorneys if psychiatric or legal problems are causing distress and thus exacerbating the patient's suffering. To that end, some hospitals and health centers have formal medical–legal partnerships through which lawyers work directly with their patients to resolve problems related to housing, custody, public assistance programs, and other matters.[22] The palliative care team can include nurses, social workers, pharmacists, chaplains, physical therapists, dieticians, and volunteers.[23] Patients who receive early palliative care for serious diseases have better outcomes even with less aggressive treatment. In one study involving 151 patients with advanced lung cancer, those receiving early palliative care scored 6.5 points higher on assessments of mood and quality of life.* In addition, their median survival was 11.6 months compared to 8.9 months for those receiving standard care, even though fewer of the palliative care patients† received aggressive end-of-life treatment.[24]

According to the National Hospice and Palliative Care Organization, approximately 5,800 hospice programs were in operation in 2013, serving between 1.5 and 1.6 million patients.[25] Roughly 50 percent of deaths involve hospice care, if only for a few days.[26] In addition, it is estimated that 80 percent of hospitals with 50 or more beds have palliative care programs.[27]

Hospice services are provided primarily in patients' homes, though they can also be provided in nursing homes, assisted living facilities, free-standing hospices, and hospitals. Medicare will pay for hospice-related medical expenses, including five days of respite care at a Medicare-approved inpatient facility in order to give the patient's usual caregiver (e.g., a family member) a break. However, Medicare will not reimburse for curative treatments, room and board, or emergency room and inpatient care unless it is arranged by the hospice team or is unrelated to the patient's terminal illness.[28] Medicare recipients who spend time in residence at a hospice facility must be prepared to pay a daily rate to cover room and board. Patients also retain the right to leave hospice and resume treatment at any time.

My first exposure to hospice came when my mother (Eema in Hebrew) spent the last two days of her life at an inpatient hospice facility. After we learned that she had advanced pancreatic cancer, we were told that if we wanted to pursue treatment, the doctors would need to intubate her and use a ventilator because she was experiencing respiratory failure. The attending physician advised us to consider giving her only comfort care. We had no difficulty deciding to follow this advice and spare Eema further torments.

The next day, we were asked to meet with the palliative care team, which consisted of a nurse and social worker. We were told that Eema could not stay in the intensive care unit now that no curative treatment was being given, a fact that we found startling and disconcerting, though it makes perfect sense in hindsight.

Eema's private hospice room was small, though in addition to the bed, it had enough chairs to seat her five family members. Other rooms appeared to

---

*Their mean score was 98.0 vs. 91.5 on a scale of 0 to 136.
†Thirty-three percent of palliative care patients received aggressive end-of-life treatment compared to 54 percent of other patients.

be larger and well decorated and presumably belonged to longer-term patients. We especially appreciated the spaces with sofas that could be reserved by family members who wanted to sleep at the hospice. Two of my sisters slept there on both nights of Eema's stay.

The nursing staff was attentive, appearing almost instantly when we pressed the call button, and frequently checked on Eema on their own. Eema received oxygen to ease her breathing and was given pain and antianxiety medications. She had no monitors and no food or water because she could not eat or drink on her own. Although she was semiconscious and at times agitated during the first evening and night, she fell into a deep sleep the next morning and seemed at peace for her last 24 hours. When she died mid-morning the following day, the staff members treated us with respect and sensitivity. Several days later, they sent a condolence card in which each wrote a personal note. They also offered my father grief counseling for several months.

A year later, my husband and I were equally impressed by the devoted care my mother-in-law received during the last six weeks of her life at a hospice unit in a Veterans' Administration hospital (she had been a woman marine during World War II). My father too spent his last three months in hospice care, though he remained at home for all but the last three days of his life. A highly competent and compassionate hospice nurse visited him twice a week, and hospice provided medical equipment, such as a hospital bed, wheelchair, and oxygen tanks. Hospice providers also came to his home to bathe him and cut his hair and nails, and on-call nurses were available 24 hours every day of the week. At the end, when his needs became too great, he was transferred to the same inpatient facility that had served my mother and received the same high quality care in his final days.

Nevertheless, hospices, like all service providers, can vary in quality. A *Washington Post* analysis published in December 2014 concluded that "[o]n several key measures, for-profit hospices as a group fall short of those run by nonprofit organizations."[29] If time permits, you should research potential hospices and select one that is highly reputable.

DIRECTING ONE'S OWN MEDICAL CARE

There are many ways for patients to exert control over their end-of-life treatment beyond entering hospice or selecting physician-assisted suicide. All patients are empowered to make choices about their medical care. Patients who are doubtful about the advice they are being given can seek a second opinion from a different doctor. And every patient with decision-making capacity has an absolute right to refuse unwanted treatment even if doing so will expedite death. This prerogative rises to the level of a constitutional right that was confirmed by the U.S. Supreme Court in the 1990 case *Cruzan v. Director, Missouri Dept. of Health.*[30]

The Problem of Overtreatment

The contemporary norm is to battle disease forcefully until the patient's last breath. This trend generates high end-of-life care costs. One study showed that Medicare expenditures in the last six months of life can reach nearly $400,000, with a median of $22,407.[31] Another source found that Medicare payments in the last year of life average $24,000 to $28,000. They account for nearly a third of all Medicare costs for seniors and 10 percent of the U.S. health care budget.[32] The study notes that these percentage figures are comparable to those in the Netherlands, where 26 percent of all spending is attributable to caring for the elderly in the last year of life but are higher than in Switzerland, where the number is reportedly 18 percent. Medicare spending declines when people die at older ages* because those who are the most elderly receive a lower intensity of care.[33] Furthermore, Medicare payments do not reflect the entire cost of treatment; they are generally supplemented by private insurance or out-of-pocket payments that can total thousands of dollars.[34] There is also significant regional variability in costs. In 2008, Dartmouth researchers examined costs for seniors with serious chronic illnesses during their last two years of life. At the Mayo Clinic in Minnesota, the costs were more than $53,000 per patient, but at the University of California–Los Angeles and New York University hospitals, they were $93,000 and $105,000, respectively.[35]

Today, there are mounting objections to the traditional approach of treating medical problems aggressively even at the end of life. In the book *Overtreated: Why Too Much Medicine Is Making Us Sicker and Poorer,* Shannon Brownlee decries the "medicalization of aging" and deems it to be "elder abuse."[36] She observes that patients and doctors tend to see "the inevitable breakdown of the body as a series of treatable diseases," which at times leads literally to torturing the dying. The author tells of one hospitalized lung cancer patient who clearly had only days to live. Yet he was subjected to the placement of a painful nasogastric feeding tube in his nose because he refused food and was tied to the bed with restraints at his wrists and ankles because he was thrashing and likely to pull out the nasogastric tube. The staff had prioritized the futile continuation of nutrition over allowing the man to spend his last days in dignity and comfort.[37]

In an autobiographical account, Michael Wolff describes his mother's travails in a moving article titled "A Life Worth Ending."[38] When his mother

---

*Medicare spends twice as much on people who die when they are 65 to 74 years old than on those dying at 85 or older.

suffered a worsening of her aortic stenosis (narrowing of the aortic valve), doctors recommended surgery. The author reports that it never occurred to him and his siblings to ask: "You want to do major heart surgery on an 84-year-old woman showing progressive signs of dementia? What are you, nuts?" According to at least some experts, general anesthesia and major surgery (especially cardiac operations) are frequently associated with the deterioration of cognitive abilities.[39]

The operation successfully repaired Mrs. Wolff's heart and added years to her life. But here is the real outcome:

> Where before she had been gently sinking [mentally], now we were in free fall. She was reduced to a terrified creature—losing language skills by the minute. . . . Unmoored in time, she began to wander the halls and was returned on regular occasions to the emergency room: Each return, each ambulance, each set of restraints, each catheter, dealt her another psychic blow.[40]

Jonathan Rauch adds his clear and strong voice of protest in the article "How Not to Die," published in the *Atlantic*. The author decries "the war on death," which he attributes to the American medical system's often unreasonable "determination to save lives" and its astonishing ability to do so through "technological virtuosity." He writes:

> Unwanted treatment is American medicine's dark continent. No one knows its extent, and few people want to talk about it. The U.S. medical system was built to treat anything that might be treatable, at any stage of life—even near the end, when there is no hope of a cure, and when the patient, if fully informed, might prefer quality time and relative normalcy to all-out intervention.[41]

Notably, a large study of nurses in Hong Kong, Ireland, Israel, Italy, and the United States revealed that the majority of nurses in all five countries would choose less aggressive treatments for themselves and their parents than they would choose for patients whose wishes were unknown. The researchers derived these findings by administering surveys to more than 1,000 nurses using hypothetical clinical case scenarios.[42] Thus, medical professionals often subject patients to treatments that they would never want for themselves or their families.

Happily, not all doctors are overly aggressive in treating the ailments of the elderly. Five months before she died of other causes, Eema learned that she had a small and slow-growing kidney cancer. We consulted top-notch experts in Ann Arbor, Michigan, and at the Cleveland Clinic, and they advised against surgery because of her advanced age and several risk factors (low kidney function, high blood pressure, heart problems). It was difficult for Eema, a long-time breast cancer survivor, to adjust to the idea that this time she would not be battling her cancer but rather, coexisting with it. Yet our family was comfortable with the decision, and believed Eema was fortunate to have seen skilled doctors who focused on what was best for her overall and spared her needless suffering.

It is also true that some doctors may embrace the approach of providing solely palliative care too quickly or be unjustifiably reluctant to provide wanted interventions to the elderly. One friend told me that her mother, who was diagnosed with cancer over a year earlier, was hospitalized in the intensive care unit. When the doctors observed that the patient was refusing food, they interpreted this as a sign that she no longer wanted to live and urged my friend "to let her go." The daughter pointed out that her mother was saying that it hurt too much to eat, which was entirely possible because she had severe chemotherapy-related mouth sores. After appropriate treatment to alleviate the symptoms, the patient began eating again. Along the same lines, in a short article published in the *Journal of the American Medical Association*, a medical student tells of her grandmother's hip replacement at the age of 90. Although physicians were hesitant to operate and urged her to accept her pain and mobility limitations, the elderly woman insisted on having the arduous operation. The author proudly relates that just 12 weeks after surgery, her grandmother "strolled, though at a slow pace, into her surgeon's office . . . with the use of no walking aids."[43]

The Power to Choose

Given alternatives and a doctor who is willing to provide care, the choice of what treatment route to follow is ultimately up to the patient or his or her health care proxy. Elderly patients can opt for aggressive interventions in an effort to prolong life or to enhance its quality. They also have a right to decline standard therapies if they wish to hasten death. For example, many patients find dialysis to be a difficult treatment, and some opt to discontinue or never start it because death from renal failure can be relatively peaceful and painless.[44] The key is for the patient or his or her proxy to understand the risks and implications of the procedure being considered and the long-term prognosis both with and without treatment.

Chapter 6, which addressed geriatric care, emphasized the importance of doing one's research before, during, and after medical encounters. This point needs to be reiterated here. Patients should not be reluctant to search the Internet for reliable sources concerning their conditions and potential treatments. Then, they should not hesitate to question their doctors about their recommendations and what is best overall in the long term. Likewise, in discussing the topic of durable power of attorney for health care in

Chapter 4, I elaborated on the need to have extensive discussions with your agent concerning end-of-life care. Do you want aggressive treatment even in the face of irreversible mental deterioration? Would you ever want to be put on a ventilator? Do you want measures that will prolong life at the expense of quality of life? If you are terminally ill, do you want family members to call an ambulance in the event of a medical crisis or do you wish to avoid hospital treatment and die at home?

Even the most well-intentioned substitute decision makers can make mistakes. Michael Wolff notes painfully that his mother's "wishes ha[d] always been properly expressed, volubly and in writing: She urgently did not want to end up where she ultimately has ended up."[45] And he acknowledges that the family did not question the doctor who suggested cardiac surgery about its implications for his mother's deteriorating mental capacities. Thus, you must make sure that your health care agent is prepared to do both of the following: (1) think carefully about what your wishes would be under the circumstances and (2) research suggested interventions and question clinicians to determine which option will best comply with your wishes.

One more set of mechanisms exists to exert control over the dying process. These are do not resuscitate (DNR) orders, out-of-hospital DNRs, and physician orders for life-sustaining treatment (POLST).

DNRs, Out-of-Hospital DNRs, and POLST

Although advance directives are created and signed by patients, DNRs, out-of-hospital DNRs, and POLST are prepared by physicians after speaking with patients or their agents. DNR orders apply in hospitals and nursing homes in limited circumstances. They instruct that the patient should not be resuscitated if his or her heart stops. Out-of-hospital DNRs are recognized in most states and are portable orders that follow the patient wherever he or she goes. The patient wears an identification tag indicating that he or she does not wish to be resuscitated by emergency personnel. POLST, which are accepted in the majority of states,[46] are medical orders that are more comprehensive than DNRs, covering not only cardiopulmonary resuscitation, but also decisions such as hospitalization, feeding tubes, antibiotics, and ventilation.[47]

Although DNRs provide clear instructions to caregivers, they have not escaped controversy. DNRs are designed to impact care only if the patient's heart actually stops. However, evidence suggests that patients with DNR orders are denied other therapeutic interventions because physicians tend to interpret the orders broadly as indicating that the patient generally wishes to reject aggressive treatment.[48] For example, DNR orders were found to be associated with refusal to admit patients to medical intensive care units.[49] Likewise, a study of acute heart failure patients revealed that the presence of DNR orders could influence the patients' course of treatment.[50] Consequently, some experts advise against premature placement of a DNR order. Instead, according to these experts, patients should ensure that their health care proxies have a detailed understanding of their wishes for decision-making purposes, and DNR orders should be used as a last resort, close to the time of anticipated death.[51]

POLST were first developed by clinicians at the Center for Ethics and Health Care at the Oregon State Health and Science University in the early 1990s. Advocates are enthusiastic about POLST because these orders cover a broader range of end-of-life treatments than DNRs and transform advance directives into actual physician orders. Because they are medical orders, they are more likely to be seen by treating physicians than advance directives, which are not always incorporated into the patient's chart or are not prominently placed in it, and thus POLST can promote greater adherence to patients' wishes.[52] The forms also travel with the patient, so that orders concerning end-of-life care can be followed in all care settings, not just hospitals. POLST forms that are endorsed by a variety of states can be downloaded from the Internet.* However, like DNRs, POLST forms generate concern that clinicians will take a low-intensity approach to caring for patients who have them and withhold interventions that the patient would want and did not mean to prohibit.[53]

RELIGIOUS BELIEFS

Those for whom religion is important should determine what their faith teaches about the permissibility of treatment cessation or withdrawal at the end of life. In my own religion, Judaism, the transition to comfort care is governed by the concept of *goses*. A *goses* is a moribund person, that is, a person who is dying. All rabbinical authorities agree that no further medical efforts need to be undertaken to prolong the life of one who has become a *goses*, though comfort measures must be continued. The problem is that there is considerable disagreement as to when the *goses* stage is reached. Some hold that one becomes a *goses* only when physicians believe that death is no more than 72 hours away. More liberal authorities offer a broader definition and teach that one can be deemed a *goses* as soon as a diagnosis of an incurable, terminal illness is made, even if the dying process could take a year or longer.[54] Consequently, Jews who would be guided by religious principles would benefit from conversations with their rabbis and from reading relevant sources in order to develop their own beliefs about the *goses* concept.

---

*Available at http://www.polst.org/endorsed-polst-forms/.

When we made the decision to discontinue Eema's treatment in the intensive care unit, we were all in agreement and did not struggle with its moral implications. Eema was clearly already dying—she was gasping for breath even with oxygen and had had no food or water by mouth for 10 days—and, in fact, she was gone within fewer than 72 hours. However, I know that in many cases, circumstances are more ambiguous, and disagreements can tear families apart and traumatize the patient.

For those who value religious doctrine, clarity about what one's faith teaches concerning end-of-life care can be very helpful. Moreover, postponing the study of religious medical ethics until one is in the midst of a medical crisis, urgently needing to make decisions, is unwise. As a member of a hospital ethics committee, I know that at times, patients or their families insist that their religion dictates certain decisions, but clergy from their denomination tell us that the individuals' understanding does not reflect formal religious doctrine. People who study religious teachings at leisure, without the pressures of a medical emergency, are more likely to obtain a deep understanding of the subject and to determine for themselves what they believe their faith requires of them.

CODA

Admittedly, it is difficult to anticipate our thoughts and wishes in times of crisis. Even those who adamantly assert that they would reject life-prolonging treatment if they were grievously ill may find that at the moment of decision they are far more ambivalent than they ever imagined they would be. The *New York Times Magazine* piece "A Life or Death Situation" crystallizes this point in a poignant story about bioethicist Peggy Battin and her husband, Brooke Hopkins, who became a quadriplegic after an accident in 2008 and suffered life-threatening health problems thereafter.[55] Although both were strong advocates of patient autonomy and the right to choose to end life rather than endure terrible suffering, they came back from the brink of declining further treatment several times before Brooke discontinued ventilation and died in 2013. Despite her copious writing on the subject, Battin found her theories very difficult to apply to her own personal situation.

Nevertheless, familiarity with options such as the possibility of rejecting unwanted care or requesting a DNR or POLST order can promote better decision making. Likewise, engaging in soul-searching about our preferences and, if relevant, understanding our own religious beliefs should facilitate the selection of appropriate end-of-life care.

These ideas are embraced by an emerging movement called the Conversation Project that promotes discussion of death and dying matters among loved ones in small social gatherings. In early 2014, hundreds of "Death over

Dinner" events were reportedly planned in the United States and other countries by groups of family members and close friends.[56] A significant number of Americans do not think about end-of-life issues at all. According to a 2013 Pew Research Center survey, one in four American adults, including those 75 and older, have given little to no thought to their preferences for end-of-life care.[57] The Conversation Project aims to change this trend.

Planning for aging should include preparation not only for living as an elderly person but also for the dying process. Doing so can be of great benefit both when we face the final illnesses of loved ones and, ultimately, when we face our own.

END-OF-LIFE PREPAREDNESS CHECKLIST

- Examine your religious or moral beliefs about end-of-life care.
- Understand that you have a right to refuse unwanted treatment.
- Ask for a palliative care consult if you or your loved one is experiencing significant discomfort.
- If you are ill and have significant legal problems, ask your doctor or hospital if your health care facility has a medical–legal partnership.
- Consider hospice if you (or a loved one) do not want life-prolonging treatment and are in the last six months of life according to your doctors.
- Consider requesting a DNR or out-of-hospital DNR order or POLST if you wish to limit care at the end of life.
- If you or a loved one may one day be interested in physician-assisted suicide and live in a state in which it is permissible, learn about the conditions under which it is potentially appropriate.

9

Conclusion

I began writing this book as a way to address my own anxieties about growing old without children and hoped that by writing it I would also help others. I ask myself now: Has what I have learned provided me with reassurance about planning for old age and my ability to take steps that will enhance my quality of life in later years? The answer is yes.

Admittedly, there are aspects of aging that are largely outside our control. One example is dementia, though some research indicates that even this ailment can be delayed or diminished through exercise, good diet, control of blood pressure and cholesterol, social engagement, and continued employment.[1] In my own life, my husband's Parkinson's disease has added a great deal of uncertainty because the condition's progression varies from person to person. We do not know how long he will be able to work, how severe his disabilities will become and when, what his care needs will be, and how much financial strain his care will place on us. I must accept that as much as I love planning, some of my plans may not come to fruition because of the hurdles that life will throw my way. I am also striving not to be excessively focused on the future and to shift to a greater extent to enjoying every day in the present because I don't know what tomorrow will bring.

Yet, there are many potential misfortunes, such as acute loneliness or inappropriate medical care, that might be avoided or whose impact might be lessened through forethought, preparedness, and a variety of interventions. The prospect of aging should not be bleak even for those without strong family support systems. In the words of physician, Harvard professor, and author

Muriel Gillick, "We need to see old age as neither all bad nor . . . all good, but rather not unlike adolescence or other challenging stages of life, as both."[2]

Have I begun to practice what I preach? Yes, in the process of writing this book, I did several things to initiate my own aging preparedness, and I have recommitted myself to a few good habits that I had already formed.

1. **Retirement communities:** I learned a lot about retirement communities in general and continuing care retirement communities (CCRCs) in particular and developed an interest in moving to a community setting after retirement. I visited only four CCRC facilities and did not find one that seemed like a perfect fit for me. As I grow older, I will continue to investigate CCRCs and other, less expensive options. I know several people who, prior to retirement, spent a week of vacation every year traveling to retirement communities in different locations. I now understand why and know that we too will need to spend considerable time at any facility that is of real interest to us.

2. **Legal documents:** I revisited and updated my will, advance directive, durable power of attorney for finances and property, and durable power of attorney for health care. I made sure that my agent (my husband) and substitute agent (my sister) have copies of my documents and I talked with them about my wishes should I become unable to make decisions for myself. I will make sure to initiate similar conversations periodically in the future.

3. **Savings and financial management:** I have always been committed to saving as much as possible. I will now continue to do so with renewed purpose, having learned much more about the cost of a comfortable retirement. I have long used financial advisers, some of whom were more helpful than others. I am pleased with our current financial advisers and will continue to consult them. My parents had periodically urged me to purchase long-term care insurance. I was glad to have the opportunity to study this product, although I decided to postpone making a decision about purchasing it. Unfortunately, I also learned that my husband became ineligible for long-term care insurance upon being diagnosed with Parkinson's disease, so it is out of the question for him.

4. **Diet and exercise:** I have exercised regularly for years and don't feel that I need to change my routine in this area. Diet is a different story. I love sweets and do not love vegetables. Am I likely to change my eating habits? Sure, but maybe not until next year!

5. **Social interaction:** My research emphasized to me the importance of having a large network of friends and relatives. Social engagement has numerous psychological and other health benefits.[3] Unfortunately, I tend to prioritize work over socializing, and I need to improve in this regard. I have tried harder to stay in touch with friends and to get

together regularly with those who live nearby. I also have made more of an effort to contact people I know when I travel to other cities and to make sure I see them and renew or maintain old friendships.

6. **Intellectual pursuits:** My work occupies my mind too much of the time, and I am trying to devote more effort to developing other intellectual interests, hobbies, and volunteer work that will sustain me after retirement. I enjoy taking nonwork-related continuing education classes and attending public lectures, reading, going to movies and the theater, being active in my synagogue, and serving as a member of a hospital ethics committee. Still, my leisure life needs improvement, and I will work on cultivating it in the future.

7. **Medical care:** As someone who had major surgery at a young age, I tend to become quite concerned about any unusual symptoms and to seek the care of specialists. As I age and my health problems become more numerous, I need to worry more about coordinated care and to take greater initiative to become a member of my own medical team. I now try routinely to ask about drug–drug interactions, side effects, and whether treatment is actually necessary. In addition, I often prepare for medical appointments by looking at reliable Internet sources. Finally, as much as I am inclined to trust the expertise of doctors, I keep in mind that I am empowered to decline unwanted treatments, seek second opinions, and not return to doctors with whom I am dissatisfied.

All in all, writing this book has provided me with reassurance. There are already many resources available to the elderly, although finding and using them may require effort. As the large population of baby boomers ages, the number and types of resources will hopefully increase considerably.

HELP FROM THE GOVERNMENT

To what extent can American seniors count on the government to provide them with needed support in old age? We are fortunate in this country to have several public safety net programs for the elderly, although I would argue that they do not go far enough. Most retirees qualify for social security payments, which depend on their earnings and how much they paid into the system.[4] Medicare covers some but not all medical expenses for those who are 65 and older, and Medicaid provides additional coverage for low-income seniors, including for nursing home care.

In addition, the Older Americans Act of 1965 (OAA)[5] helps fund the delivery of certain social services to the aging population.[6] The law established the Administration on Aging within the Department of Health and

Human Services and provides for grants that support state, local, and private agencies furnishing services such as meals, transportation, home care, aid for family caregivers, and disease prevention and health promotion programs. However, in 2014, OAA funding totaled only 1.9 billion,[7] which meant that only approximately 5 percent of eligible adults (those 60 and older) benefited regularly from OAA-funded programs, and 14 percent benefited intermittently.[8]

By contrast, the governments of some countries play a more proactive role in ensuring the welfare of their elderly. Not surprisingly, these countries often have higher tax rates than we do in the United States. For example, Sweden's Social Services Act establishes that people of all ages have a right to receive services if their needs cannot otherwise be met. Swedish municipalities offer meals that are home delivered or available at adult daycare centers whose cost varies with income. The government provides public and special transportation services that are accessible to individuals with disabilities. Home care assistance is also widely available at fees that are calculated based on household income and living expenses. Informal caregivers, such as family members, can also obtain payment in the form of a "carer's allowance" and four hours of cost-free respite coverage per week. Services are offered through either a public provider or a private company subsidized by the government.[9]

Given our aversion to high taxes, it is unlikely that the U.S. government will significantly increase funding for programs or services in the foreseeable future. Nevertheless, many charitable organizations, religious institutions, and private enterprises offer a wealth of services and programs for seniors.

What the Future Holds

The resources that I have described in these chapters are already available to seniors. The future, however, promises to bring support mechanisms that are only in the earliest stages of development today.

Technology may significantly extend seniors' ability to remain independent and mobile. For example, as discussed in Chapter 5, autonomous cars may enable elderly individuals to drive even in the face of impairments that would otherwise affect their reaction time and driving ability.[10] Similarly, robots may help elderly individuals with various tasks and allow them to continue living at home.[11]

Entrepreneurs are also creating technology for "smart homes." These include a large number of safety and comfort-enhancing features:

- Motion-detecting cameras and ultrasonic location tracking devices;
- Blinds that close automatically when the air conditioning is on to reduce the need for cooling;

- Smart floors with embedded pressure sensors and chair sensors to detect falls and report them to emergency services;
- Mailboxes that notify residents when mail arrives;
- Beds that monitor sleeping patterns;
- Mirrors that display messages such as medication reminders;
- Toilets that track changes in voiding habits;
- Water monitors to detect leaks or overflows;
- Showers that automatically regulate water temperature;
- Temperature monitors that send alerts if the temperature in the home is out of normal range;
- Sensors attached to household appliances to monitor food preparation and eating.[12]

It is not clear how expensive such items will be if they are widely marketed and whether they would be affordable for people of modest means. Nevertheless, in planning for old age, we should familiarize ourselves with existing and emerging resources. Several other essential planning themes have been developed in this book and are worth highlighting here.

THE IMPORTANCE OF SOCIAL LIFE

A robust social life is critical to happiness at any time in life and especially after retirement, when people no longer interact with others through work on a daily basis. The elderly are vulnerable to becoming socially isolated for a variety of reasons. They may no longer be able to travel to visit loved ones. They may withdraw from social, civic, or intellectual activities because of disability or transportation challenges. They may have difficulty communicating with others and participating in conversations because of hearing impairment. They may become housebound because of severe mobility or cognitive impairments. And they may not have visitors because their contemporaries are frail or predecease them. At the same time, seniors cherish their autonomy and often prioritize "aging in place" and continuing to live independently in their longtime homes, no matter how lonely or disabled they are.

This approach, however, is ill conceived. In the words of Dr. Muriel Gillick, a geriatric specialist, "baby boomers will need to give up our single-minded devotion to individual autonomy and to accept the fact that community is tremendously important as we age."[13]

Baby boomers should seriously consider moving to retirement communities while they are robust enough to enjoy their offerings. Such facilities foster social integration and furnish safe and accessible homes for the elderly. Aging within a close and vibrant community is of far greater value than aging in a home that is spacious and holds memories of decades past.

All of us should emphasize nurturing friendships and expanding our social circles throughout life. Involvement in a church, synagogue, mosque, or other religious entity often provides a natural mechanism for social contact, as does membership in other organizations. Do not give up opportunities to meet new people, see friends, and build a network of people to care about.

RETAINING A SENSE OF PURPOSE AND USEFULNESS

To be happy, you need not only friends but also meaning and purpose in life. After retirement, career must be replaced by other rewarding activities, such as volunteer work, a creative outlet, or advocacy for a good cause.

Several months after he was widowed, my father wrote a short memoir and reported that this undertaking gave him a "renewed appetite for life." Other acquaintances donate their time to charitable organizations, take classes, become politically active, and develop their artistic talents in areas such as painting or photography, to which they could devote only minimal time in the past. Younger retirees could also contribute to the well-being of older seniors by assisting them with driving, errands, and household chores either as volunteers or for a modest fee.

Some who need income or enjoy having jobs seek part-time work, not always in a field that is related to their prior careers. Like volunteer work and leisure activities, so-called bridge work has been found to be strongly related to life satisfaction after retirement.[14]

Involvement in nonjob-related activities should not be postponed until old age, when it might be difficult to undertake completely new initiatives. To prepare for retirement, therefore, middle-aged individuals should cultivate hobbies, interests, and volunteer work that they can continue to pursue later in life.

WRITE YOUR LEGISLATOR

Baby boomers have a strong political voice and are a vital economic force in the United States. We should use these advantages to advocate for ourselves and persuade policymakers to address the needs of elderly members of society.

Approximately 77 million Americans were born between 1946 and 1964, and thus baby boomers constituted 26 percent of the population in 2010.[15] Baby boomers' annual spending power is $2.2 trillion, and we have achieved higher levels of education than any prior generation.[16] Baby boomers represent 37 percent of registered voters, exceeding any other generation.[17] Seniors themselves are known to be active voters, and political candidates invest considerable effort in courting them. In the 2012 presidential election, 72 percent of individuals who were 65 and older voted, compared with 59 percent of the general eligible electorate.[18]

The elderly in this country experience many challenges, and many of these are not likely to be alleviated in the near future. We face the threat of significant cuts to Medicare and social security benefits, insufficient savings, very costly long-term care insurance, a dearth of accessible transportation options, and a scarcity of geriatric and palliative care specialists, to name just a few. We must frequently remind government officials that baby boomers and seniors care deeply about these issues and press them to take action in the form of public programs and legislative solutions.

As just one example, Congress and state legislatures could implement a variety of measures to address the shortage of primary care and geriatric physicians. More generous Medicare reimbursement for geriatric services would be an obvious way to increase the attractiveness of the field. The same is true of loan forgiveness programs, scholarships, and other financial incentives for medical students. More extensive requirements for education about elder care in medical school and for licensure and certification purposes would also be of benefit.[19] Already, the Patient Protection and Affordable Care Act ("Obamacare") established a program that will operate through 2015 by which primary care physicians can receive a 10 percent bonus for seeing Medicare patients.[20] It also dedicated money to programs designed to help train thousands of new primary care physicians.[21] More recently, the Resident Physician Shortage Reduction Act of 2013 was introduced by Representatives Joseph Crowley (D-NY) and Michael Grimm (R-NY) to increase the number of residency slots by 15,000 over five years, with many slots dedicated to specialties in which a shortage exists. The bill, however, was not passed.

The issues that affect seniors can become a priority if we make them so. In the words of Dr. Muriel Gillick, "our voices matter, although we may need to speak in unison to be heard."[22]

REMAIN ADEPT AT USING TECHNOLOGY

Technology is evolving at a dizzying pace, and it is at times frustrating and difficult to keep up with its many changes. Although I use computers every day, when I bought a new laptop that had Windows 8 instead of Windows 7, I could barely operate it, and even my computer-scientist husband was initially baffled. We had to call a friend who is a software engineer for a personal tutoring lesson.

Nevertheless, technology is just as important for the old as it is for the young. Elderly people who are sophisticated about e-mail and the Internet are less likely to become the victims of scams and fraudulent schemes that target the naive and gullible.

In addition, patients increasingly rely on computers and electronic devices for their health needs. Electronic personal health records allow patients to view test results, appointment schedules, and other information in their medical records. Using the Internet, patients can research their symptoms, treatments, and medical conditions prior to seeing their physicians or obtain additional information after a doctor's visit. Telehealth enables clinicians to monitor physiological health data remotely so that patients need not come to the clinic as frequently. Electronic medication dispensers can provide timed reminders, monitoring, and alerts to caregivers when medications are forgotten or taken improperly.

Technology can also promote the social, intellectual, and physical fitness of the elderly. E-mail, Facebook, and Skype enable individuals to remain in close contact with friends and relatives who live far away. Hobby forums, online courses, and many other offerings create opportunities for intellectual engagement. Wii games enable seniors to exercise their bodies and minds in their own living rooms.[23]

As we age, we should continue to embrace technology and remain updated about its uses and evolution. Even the very old should feel comfortable navigating a computer and using sophisticated technological devices. The first generation iPhone was released only in 2007, and now many millions of people worldwide cannot conceive of life without it. We cannot even begin to imagine what the future will bring us. To enjoy the benefits of communication, entertainment, and information, we must not allow our technology skills to atrophy no matter how old we are.

A FINAL PREPAREDNESS CHECKLIST

I have provided checklists at the end of each chapter. Now, I will further streamline the primary points of *Aging with a Plan* into a single preparedness checklist. Here is what you can do in middle age to prepare for old age:

- Save as much money as possible for retirement. Do not underestimate your expenses or how much money you will need after you stop working.
- If possible, obtain financial advice from professional experts.
- Prepare legal documents: a will and possibly a trust, a living will, a durable power of attorney for finances and property, a durable power of attorney for health care, an anatomical gift form if desired, and, if relevant, an advance directive for mental health treatment.
- Have periodic conversations with your agents for health care and financial matters concerning your wishes regarding finances, medical treatment, and end-of-life care should you become incapacitated.

- Supplement your will with a list of valuables, such as jewelry and cars, indicating to whom they should be distributed upon death. This list should be updated periodically and accessible to the executor of your estate or trustee. Also, create a list that explains where important financial documents and items can be found (e.g., drawers at home, a safe, a safe deposit box in a bank) and give it to your agent for financial matters and the alternate. Provide instructions as to your preferred funeral and burial or cremation arrangements.
- Exercise regularly and maintain a healthy diet in order to prevent, delay, and diminish the impact of health problems in old age.
- Become a sophisticated user of technology.
- Learn about resources, such as senior centers and transportation options, that are available to the elderly and about professionals, such as daily money managers and geriatric care managers, that can provide assistance.
- Begin to explore retirement communities such as CCRCs. Recognize that "aging in place" can have significant disadvantages in terms of social isolation and boredom.
- Accept the fact that you may not be able to drive forever and commit to stopping on your own before you become an unsafe driver.
- As you age, pay special attention to safety features and safety-oriented technology when purchasing automobiles.
- Find a good primary care physician and pursue appropriate preventive care. Plan to see a geriatric specialist if you develop multiple, complicated health problems when you are elderly.
- Develop good habits as a patient that will persist into old age. Become an active member of your own medical team. Do research, ask questions, and seek second opinions when you are uncertain about which option is best.
- Do not make important medical decisions or undergo serious treatments alone. Have a close friend or relative accompany you, and hire aides when you require extra support at home or in the hospital.
- Determine what your moral beliefs are concerning end-of-life care. Read ethics literature and study religious doctrine, if it is meaningful for you.
- Keep the option of hospice in mind. It is a legal and widely available way to transition from aggressive treatment of a terminal illness to comfort care that can alleviate suffering at the end of life.
- Nurture strong friendships and relationships with family members, pursue hobbies, and become involved in volunteer work.
- Dream about retirement and plan for it to be life-enriching and fulfilling.

Despite being a workaholic, I look forward to retirement and imagine a variety of activities that will make me happy. I think about studying to be a docent at an art museum and then using my teaching skills to serve as a tour guide for museum visitors. I look forward to attending courses, lectures, and the theater. I will continue to exercise regularly and volunteer, perhaps at a hospital. I will frequently get together with friends and dream of traveling a lot if our finances and my husband's health permit us to do so. I will keep busy but make time to relax, and I will not write articles or books!

Baby boomers are reluctant to think about our own old age, much less plan for it.[24] We often watch our elderly relatives suffer, we shudder, and we fervently hope that we will be able to avoid a similar fate. Nevertheless, we might be able to help our loved ones avoid some of their anguish by having conversations with them about difficult topics such as moving to an appropriate residential setting, driving, and end-of-life care long before they need to make immediate decisions in a crisis. And surely we can help ourselves by planning ahead. Having a high quality of life in old age requires effort and forethought, especially for those of us who will not have a strong family support network. The good news is that however unpredictable the aging process may be, it need not be left entirely in the hands of destiny. We can take the initiative to remain active physically, mentally, and socially and implement antidotes to isolation and depression. Having done my research and written this book, I'm reassured about our prospects as seniors. Armed with information and a plan, we can do much to direct our future and achieve a high quality of life no matter how old we are.

Notes

INTRODUCTION

1. June R. Lunney, Joanne Lynn, and Christopher Hogan, "Profiles of Older Medicare Decedents," *Journal of the American Geriatrics Society* 50, no. 6 (2002): 1110 (classifying the other patients as having died because of terminal illness [22 percent], organ system failure [16 percent], frailty [47 percent], or other causes); June R. Lunney et al., "Patterns of Functional Decline at the End of Life," *Journal of the American Medical Association* 289, no. 18 (May 2003): 2389 (categorizing the remaining individuals as dying of cancer [21 percent], organ failure [20 percent], frailty [20 percent], and other causes [24 percent]).

2. Sandra L. Colby and Jennifer M. Ortman, "The Baby Boom Cohort in the United States: 2012 to 2060: Population Estimates and Projections," *United States Census Bureau Report* P25-1141, May 2014, 15, accessed November 7, 2014, http://www.census.gov/prod/2014pubs/p25-1141.pdf.

3. "Population," Federal Interagency Forum on Aging Related Statistics, accessed October 16, 2014, http://www.agingstats.gov/Main_Site/Data/2012_Documents/Population.aspx.

4. Jennifer M. Ortman, Victoria A. Velkoff, and Howard Hogan, "An Aging Nation: The Older Population in the United States: Population Estimates and Projections," *United States Census Bureau Report* P25-1140, May 2014, 6, accessed November 7, 2014, https://www.census.gov/content/dam/Census/library/publications/2014/demo/p25-1140.pdf.

5. Jiaquan Xu et al., "Mortality in the United States, 2012," *NCHS Data Brief* no. 168 (October 2014), 1, accessed November 10, 2014, http://www.cdc.gov/nchs/data/databriefs/db168.pdf.

6. Maggie Koerth-Baker, "Death of a Caveman: What Swedish Babies and the Stone Age Can Teach Us About Life Expectancy and Income Inequality," *New York Times Magazine*, March 24, 2013, 14.

7. Lawrence A. Frolik and Linda S. Whitton, *Everyday Law for Seniors: Updated with the Latest Federal Benefits* (Boulder, CO: Paradigm Publishers, 2012), 3.

8. Virginia M. Freid, Amy B. Bernstein, and Mary Ann Bush, "Multiple Chronic Conditions Among Adults Aged 45 and Over: Trends Over the Past 10 Years," *NCHS Data Brief* no. 100 (July 2012), 1, accessed October 16, 2014, http://www.cdc.gov/nchs/data/databriefs/db100.pdf.

9. "2014 Alzheimer's Disease Facts and Figures," Alzheimer's Association, 16, accessed November 10, 2014, http://www.alz.org/downloads /Facts_Figures_2014.pdf. This resource estimates that in 2014, 5.2 million Americans had Alzheimer's disease. Thus, 11 percent of individuals 65 and older were Alzheimer's patients, and the figure rose to 32 percent for those 85 and over. Moreover, 13.9 percent of those 71 and older have some form of dementia, which is a broad category of mental impairments that extends well beyond Alzheimer's disease.

10. Fiona E. Matthews et al., "A Two-Decade Comparison of Prevalence of Dementia in Individuals Aged 65 Years and Older from Three Geographical Areas of England: Results of the Cognitive Function and Ageing Study I and II," *Lancet* 382, no. 9902 (2013): 1405, accessed October 16, 2014, http://download.thelancet.com/flatcontentassets/pdfs/S0140673613615706 .pdf.

11. Kaare Christensen et al., "Physical and Cognitive Functioning of People Older than 90 Years: A Comparison of Two Danish Cohorts Born 10 Years Apart," *Lancet* 382, no. 9903 (2013): 1509; Eric B. Larson, Kristine Yaffe, and Kenneth M. Langa, "New Insights into the Dementia Epidemic," *New England Journal of Medicine* 369 (2013): 2275.

12. Gina Kolata, "Dementia Rate Is Found to Drop Sharply, as Forecast," *New York Times*, June 16, 2013, accessed October 16, 2014, http://www .nytimes.com/2013/07/17/health/study-finds-dip-in-dementia-rates.html? _r=0.

13. Muriel R. Gillick, *The Denial of Aging: Perpetual Youth, Eternal Life, and Other Dangerous Fantasies* (Cambridge, MA: Harvard University Press, 2006), 257–58; T. Vogel et al., "Health Benefits of Physical Activity in Older Patients: A Review," *International Journal of Clinical Practice* 63, no. 2 (2009): 304–15; Mayo Clinic Staff, "Mediterranean Diet: A Heart-Healthy Eating Plan," Mayo Clinic, accessed October 16, 2014, http://www.mayoclinic .com/health/mediterranean-diet/CL00011.

14. "2014 Alzheimer's Disease Facts and Figures," 43.

15. "2014 Alzheimer's Disease Facts and Figures," 35–36.

16. "Population," Federal Interagency Forum on Aging Related Statistics.

17. "A Profile of Older Americans: 2013," U.S. Department of Health and Human Services Administration on Aging & Administration for Community Living, 1, accessed November 10, 2014, http://www.aoa.acl.gov /Aging_Statistics/Profile/2013/docs/2013_Profile.pdf.

18. "2014 Alzheimer's Disease Facts and Figures," 48.

19. Lindsay M. Monte and Renee R. Ellis, "Fertility of Women in the United States: 2012," *United States Census Population Characteristics* P20-575, July 2014, 5, accessed November 10, 2014, http://www.census.gov/content /dam/Census/library/publications/2014/demo/p20-575.pdf.

20. Irene M. Thomas, "Childless by Choice: Why Some Latinas Are Saying No to Motherhood," *Hispanic* 8, no. 4 (May 1995): 50.

21. Organisation for Economic Co-operation and Development, *The Future of Families to 2030* (OECD Publishing, 2012), 20, accessed October 16, 2014, http://www.leavenetwork.org/fileadmin/Leavenetwork/News /Future_Families_2030.pdf,

22. Joan Didion, *Blue Nights* (New York: Vintage, 2011), 185.

CHAPTER 1

1. "Retirement Calculator: Full Retirement Age," U.S. Social Security Administration, accessed October 16, 2014, http://www.ssa.gov/retire2 /retirechart.htm.

2. Neil Shah, "More Young Adults Live with Parents," *Wall Street Journal*, August 27, 2013, accessed October 16, 2014, http://online.wsj.com/news /articles/SB10001424127887324906304579039313087064716.

3. "10 Percent of Grandparents Live with a Grandchild, Census Bureau Reports," *United States Census Bureau News Release*, no. CB 14-194, October 22, 2014, accessed October 22, 2014, http://www.census.gov /newsroom/press-releases/2014/cb14-194.html.

4. Kim Parker and Eileen Patten, "The Sandwich Generation: Rising Financial Burdens for Middle-Aged Americans," *Pew Research Center Social & Demographic Trends*, January 30, 2013, accessed October 16, 2014, http:// www.pewsocialtrends.org/2013/01/30/the-sandwich-generation/.

5. Ruth Helman, Craig Copeland, and Jack VanDerhei, "The 2012 Retirement Confidence Survey: Job Insecurity, Debt Weigh on Retirement, Confidence, Savings," *Employee Benefit Research Institute Brief* 369 (2012), 5, accessed October 16, 2014, http://www.ebri.org/pdf/surveys /rcs/2012/EBRI_IB_03-2012_No369_RCS.pdf.

6. "Most Middle-Income Workers Saving Less Than Five Percent of Their Income for Retirement," *LIMRA*, October 31, 2012, accessed October 16, 2014, http://www.limra.com/Posts/PR/News_Releases/Most_Middle -Income_Workers_Saving_Less_Than_Five_Percent_of_Their_Income _for_Retirement.aspx.

7. "Fact Sheet: Social Security," U.S. Social Security Administration, 1, accessed October 16, 2014, http://www.ssa.gov/pressoffice/factsheets /basicfact-alt.pdf. The 2014 Retirement Confidence Survey conducted by the Employee Benefit Research Institute likewise found that 36 percent of respondents stated that they have less than $1,000 in savings. Ruth Helman et al., "The 2014 Retirement Confidence Survey: Confidence Rebounds— for Those with Retirement Plans," *Employee Benefit Research Institute Brief* 397 (2014), 5, accessed October 23, 2014, http://www.ebri.org/pdf /briefspdf/EBRI_IB_397_Mar14.RCS.pdf.

8. Richard W. Johnson and Corina Mommaerts, The Urban Institute, *Will Healthcare Costs Bankrupt Aging Boomers?* (Washington, DC: Urban Institute, 2010), 11, accessed October 23, 2014, http://www.urban.org /uploadedpdf/412026_health_care_costs.pdf; Allison K. Hoffman and Howell E. Jackson, "Retiree Out-of-Pocket Healthcare Spending: A Study of Consumer Expectations and Policy Implications," *American Journal of Law and Medicine* 39, no. 1 (2013): 12.

9. Ashlee Vance, "Why Do Hearing Aids Cost More Than Laptops?," *Bloomberg Businessweek Technology*, June 6, 2013, accessed October 16, 2014, http://www.businessweek.com/articles/2013-06-06/why-do-hearing -aids-cost-more-than-laptops; Ian Cropp, "Why Do Hearing Aids Cost So Much?," *AARP Bulletin*, May 5, 2011, accessed October 16, 2014, http://www.aarp.org/health/conditions-treatments/info-05-2011/hearing -aids-cost.html.

10. Amy S. Kelley et al., "Out-of-Pocket Spending in the Last Five Years of Life," *Journal of General Internal Medicine* 28, no. 2 (2013): 307.

11. Martha M. Hamilton, "What Health Care Will Cost You," *AARP Bulletin*, January/February 2013, accessed October 31, 2014, http://www.aarp.org /health/medicare-insurance/info-12-2012/health-care-costs.html.

12. Hoffman, "Retiree Out-of-Pocket Healthcare Spending," 67.

13. "Attitudes about Aging: A Global Perspective," *Pew Research Global Attitudes Project*, January 30, 2014, accessed October 16, 2014, http://www .pewglobal.org/2014/01/30/attitudes-about-aging-a-global-perspective/.

14. *Health Care & Retirement Corp. of America v. Pittas*, 46 A.3d 719 (Pa.Super. 2012).

15. Eve Kaplan, "New Financial Burden For Boomers: Forced to Pay Parents' Long-Term-Care Costs," *Forbes*, August 13, 2012, accessed October 16, 2014, http://www.forbes.com/sites/feeonlyplanner/2012/08/13/new-financial-burden-for-boomers-forced-to-pay-parents-long-term-care-bill/; Katherine C. Pearson, "Filial Support Laws in the Modern Era: Domestic and International Comparison of Enforcement Practices for Laws Requiring Adult Children to Support Indigent Parents," *Elder Law Journal* 20 (2013): 275–277.

16. Helman, Copeland, and VanDerhei, "The 2012 Retirement Confidence Survey."

17. Richard H. Thaler and Cass R. Sunstein, *Nudge: Improving Decisions About Health, Wealth, and Happiness* (New York: Penguin, 2009), 109.

18. See, for example, "Is Opening a Roth IRA Right for You?," Fifth Third Bank, accessed October 16, 2014, https://www.53.com/site/personal-banking /investments/our-solutions/rsp-roth-iras.html.

19. 20 C.F.R. §404.313 (2014).

20. 20 C.F.R. §404.409 (2014).

21. Ann Carrns, "Save for Retirement First, the Children's Education Second," *New York Times*, March 1, 2014, B4.

22. "Simple Savings Calculator," BankRate, accessed October 16, 2014, http://www.bankrate.com/calculators/savings/simple-savings-calculator .aspx.

23. J. D. Roth, "How Much Should You Save for Retirement?," *Time*, December 5, 2012, accessed October 16, 2014, http://business.time.com/2012/12/05 /how-much-should-you-save-for-retirement/.

24. "Simple Retirement Calculator," Moneychimp, accessed October 16, 2014, http://www.moneychimp.com/calculator/retirement_calculator .htm.

25. "Ballpark E$timate," Choose to Save, accessed October 16, 2014, http:// www.choosetosave.org/ballpark/index.cfm?fa=interactive.

26. "Pro Bono," Financial Planning Association, accessed October 16, 2014, http://www.onefpa.org/advocacy/Pages/ProBonoProgram.aspx.

27. See, for example, "FPA CT Pro Bono Network," Financial Planning Association, accessed October 16, 2014, http://fpact.org/net/home/ProBono /FpaCtProBonoNetwork.pdf); "Office of Connecticut State Treasurer Denise L. Nappier and Financial Planning Associations of Connecticut Announce the FPA CT Pro Bono Network," *Office of CT State Treasurer News*, November 10, 2008, accessed October 16, 2014, http://www.ott.ct.gov/pressreleases /press2008/PR11102008.pdf.

28. "The People and Mission Behind Wife.org," Women's Institute for Financial Education, accessed October 16, 2014, http://www.wife.org.

29. "How to Choose a Financial Planner," *Wall Street Journal*, December 17, 2008, accessed October 16, 2014, http://guides.wsj.com/personal-finance /managing-your-money/how-to-choose-a-financial-planner/tab/print/.

30. Thaler and Sunstein, *Nudge: Improving Decisions About Health, Wealth, and Happiness*, 120.

31. Steve Weisman, *A Guide to Elder Planning: Everything You Need to Know to Protect Yourself Legally and Financially* (Upper Saddle River, NJ: Prentice Hall, 2004), 76.

32. Thaler and Sunstein, *Nudge: Improving Decisions About Health, Wealth, and Happiness*, 125.

33. LearnVest, accessed October 16, 2014, https://www.learnvest.com/; Tara Siegel Bernard, "Start-Up Aims to Bring Financial Planning to the Masses," *New York Times*, July 27, 2013, B1 & B4.

34. Lauren Harris-Kojetin et al., *Long-Term Care Services in the United States: 2013 Overview* (Hyattsville, MD: National Center for Health Statistics, 2013), 2, accessed November 7, 2014, http://www.cdc.gov/nchs/data/nsltcp/long_term_care_services_2013.pdf.

35. Richard W. Johnson and Janice S. Park, "Who Purchases Long-Term Care Insurance?," *Urban Institute, Older Americans' Economic Security* 29 (March 2011), 1, accessed October 16, 2014, http://www.urban.org/UploadedPDF/412324-Long-Term-Care-Insurance.pdf; Jeffrey R. Brown and Amy Finkelstein, "Insuring Long-Term Care in the United States," *Journal of Economic Perspective* 25, no. 4 (2011): 122.

36. Brown, "Insuring Long-Term Care in the United States," 123.

37. Brown, "Insuring Long-Term Care in the United States," 124; Johnson and Park, "Who Purchases Long-Term Care Insurance?," 1.

38. Anne Kelly et al., "Length of Stay for Older Adults Residing in Nursing Homes at the End of Life," *Journal of American Geriatrics Society* 58, no. 9 (2010): 1703.

39. Brown, "Insuring Long-Term Care in the United States," 125.

40. National Association of Insurance Commissioners, *Buyer's Guide to Long-Term Care Insurance* (Kansas City, MO: National Association of Insurance Commissioners, 2013), 33.

41. Brown, "Insuring Long-Term Care in the United States," 126–127.

42. Brown, "Insuring Long-Term Care in the United States," 127–128.

43. National Association of Insurance Commissioners, *Buyer's Guide to Long-Term Care Insurance*, 28.

44. Lawrence A. Frolik and Linda S. Whitton, *Everyday Law for Seniors* (Boulder, CO: Paradigm Publishers 2012), 85–86.

45. Enid Kassner, "Private Long-Term Care Insurance: The Medicaid Interaction," *AARP Issue Brief* 68 (2004), 2–7, accessed October 16, 2014, http://assets.aarp.org/rgcenter/health/ib68_ltc.pdf.

46. Brown, "Insuring Long-Term Care in the United States," 129.

47. Brown, "Insuring Long-Term Care in the United States, 135.

48. "Secretary Sebelius' Letter to Congress about CLASS," October 14, 2011, accessed October 16, 2014, http://www.ltcconsultants.com/articles/2011/class-dismissed/Sebelius-CLASS-Letter.pdf.

49. Jeffrey R. Brown, Gopi Shah Goda, and Kathleen McGarry, "Long-Term Care Insurance Demand Limited by Beliefs about Needs, Concerns about Insurers, and Care Available from Family," *Health Affairs* 31, no. 6 (2012): 1300.

50. Kelly Greene, "Long-Term Care: What Now?," *Wall Street Journal*, March 9, 2012, accessed October 16, 2014, http://online.wsj.com/articles/SB10 001424052970203961204577269842991276650.

51. Kainaz Amaria, "Long-Term Care Insurance: Who Needs It?," *NPR Special Series Family Matters: The Money Squeeze*, May 8, 2012, accessed October 16, 2014, http://www.npr.org/2012/05/08/151970188/long-term -care-insurance-who-needs-it.

52. Howard Gleckman, "Should You Buy Long-Term Care Insurance? Maybe Not," *Forbes*, January 18, 2012, accessed October 16, 2014, http://www .forbes.com/sites/howardgleckman/2012/01/18/should-you-buy-long-term- care-insurance-maybe-not/; Emily Brandon, "The Best Age to Buy Long- Term-Care Insurance," *U.S. News*, September 2, 2008, accessed October 16, 2014, http://money.usnews.com/money/blogs/planning-to-retire/2008/09/02 /the-best-age-to-buy-long-term-care-insurance.

53. "Should You Purchase Long-Term-Care Insurance?," *Wall Street Journal*, May 14, 2012, accessed October 16, 2014, http://online.wsj.com/article /SB10001424052702303425504577352031401783756.html.

54. Greene, "Long-Term Care: What Now?"

55. Peter Kyle, "Confronting the Elder Care Crisis: The Private Long-Term Care Insurance Market and the Utility of Hybrid Products," *Marquette Elder's Advisor*, 15 (2013): 128–130.

56. Enrique Zamora, Deborah Nodar, and Krista Ogletree, "Long-Term Care Insurance: A Life Raft for Baby Boomers," *Saint Thomas Law Review*, 26 (2013): 96.

57. "Your Guide to Reverse Mortgages," National Reverse Mortgage Lenders Association, 2014, accessed October 16, 2014, http://www.reversemortgage .org/.

58. Carolyn Rosenblatt, "The Hidden Truths about Reverse Mortgages," *Forbes*, July 23, 2012, accessed October 16, 2014, http://www.forbes.com /sites/carolynrosenblatt/2012/07/23/hidden-truths-about-reverse-mortgages /2/.

CHAPTER 2

1. Gretchen Rubin, *The Happiness Project: Or, Why I Spent a Year Trying to Sing in the Morning, Clean My Closets, Fight Right, Read Aristotle, and Generally Have More Fun* (New York: HarperCollins, 2009), 142.

2. Karl Pillemer and Nina Glasgow, "Social Integration and Aging," in *Social Integration in the Second Half of Life*, ed. Karl Pillemer, Phyllis Moen, Elaine Wethington, and Nina Glasgow (Baltimore, MD: Johns Hopkins University Press, 2000), 41; George E. Vaillant, *Aging Well: Surprising Guideposts to a Happier Life from the Landmark Harvard Study of Adult Development* (Boston: Little Brown and Company, 2002), 200.

3. Carla M. Perissinotto, Irena Stijacic Cenzer, and Kenneth E. Covinsky, "Loneliness in Older Persons: A Predictor of Functional Decline and Death," *Archives of Internal Medicine* 172, no. 44 (2012): 1078.

4. Anthony D. Ong, Jeremy D. Rothstein, and Bert N. Uchino, "Loneliness Accentuates Age Differences in Cardiovascular Responses to Social Evaluative Threat," *Psychology and Aging* 27, no. 1 (2012): 196.

5. "Social Support, Networks, and Happiness," Population Reference Bureau, *Today's Research on Aging* 17 (2009): 2.

6. Karen Ertel, Maria Glymour, and Lisa F. Berkman, "Effects of Social Integration on Preserving Memory Function in a Nationally Representative US Elderly Population," *American Journal of Public Health* 98, no. 7 (2008): 1218–20; Valerie C. Crooks et al., "Social Network, Cognitive Function, and Dementia Incidence Among Elderly Women," *American Journal of Public Health* 98, no. 7 (2008): 1225.

7. Joe Tomaka, Sharon Thompson, and Rebecca Palacios, "The Relation of Social Isolation, Loneliness, and Social Support to Disease Outcomes among the Elderly," *Journal of Aging and Health* 18, no. 3 (2006): 377–381; Julianne Holt-Lunstad, Timothy B. Smith, and J. Bradley Layton, "Social Relationships and Mortality Risk: A Meta-Analytic Review," *PLoS Medicine* 7, no. 7 (2010): 14–15.

8. Ayako Morita et al., "Contribution of Interaction with Family, Friends and Neighbours, and Sense of Neighbourhood Attachment to Survival in Senior Citizens: 5-Year Follow-Up Study," *Social Science and Medicine* 70, no. 4 (2009): 546.

9. Sahab Sinha, P. Nayyar, and Surat P. Sinha, "Social Support and Self-Control as Variables in Attitude toward Life and Perceived Control among Older People in India," *Journal of Social Psychology* 142, no. 4 (2002): 534–537.

10. Katherine L. Fiori, Toni C. Antonucci, and Kai S. Cortina, "Social Network Typologies and Mental Health among Older Adults," *Journal of Gerontology: Series B* 61, no. 1 (2006): 31.

11. Tara L. Gruenewald et al., "Increased Mortality Risk in Older Adults with Persistently Low or Declining Feelings of Usefulness to Others," *Journal of Aging Health* 21, no. 2 (2009): 422. The study involved 1189 adults who were 70 to 79 years old.

12. Pillemer and Glasgow, "Social Integration and Aging," 37–38.

13. Judith Shulevitz, "Why Do Grandmothers Exist?," *The New Republic*, January 29, 2013, accessed October 20, 2014, http://www.newrepublic.com/article/112199/genetics-grandmothers-why-they-exist.

14. John Wallis Rowe and Robert Louis Kahn, *Successful Aging* (New York: Dell Publishing, 1998), 178.

15. Vaillant, *Aging Well*, 248.

16. "55+ Communities," SeniorHomes.com, accessed October 20, 2014, http://www.seniorhomes.com/p/55-communities/.

17. Paula Span, *When the Time Comes: Families with Aging Parents Share Their Struggles and Solutions* (New York: Springboard Press, 2009), 3.

18. "NORC: Georgia's Neighborhood Approach to Healthy Aging," accessed October 20, 2014, http://www.tocohillsnorc.org/.

19. Andrew Scharlach, Carrie Graham, and Amanda Lehning, "The 'Village' Model: A Consumer-Driven Approach for Aging in Place," *Gerontologist* 52, no. 3 (2011): 422.

20. See http://nationalsharedhousing.org/ and http://www.goldengirlsnet work.org/, accessed October 20, 2014.

21. Sally Abrahms, "House Sharing for Boomer Women Who Would Rather Not Live Alone," *AARP Bulletin*, May 31, 2013, accessed October 20, 2014, http://www.aarp.org/home-family/your-home/info-05-2013/older -women-roommates-house-sharing.html.

22. "Senior Centers: Fact Sheet," National Council on Aging, accessed October 20, 2014, http://www.ncoa.org/press-room/fact-sheets/senior -centers-fact-sheet.html.

23. "About MOWAA," Meals on Wheels Association of America, accessed October 20, 2014, http://www.mowaa.org/aboutus.

24. Edward A. Frongillo and Wendy S. Wolfe, "Impact of Participation in Home-Delivered Meals on Nutrient Intake, Dietary Patterns, and Food Insecurity of Older Persons in New York State," *Journal of Nutrition for the Elderly* 29, no. 3 (2010): 305–306; Edward A. Frongillo et al., "Adequacy of and Satisfaction with Delivery and Use of Home-Delivered Meals," *Journal of Nutrition for the Elderly* 29, no. 3 (2010): 222–224.

25. Elizabeth O'Brien, "Know Your Retirement Community's Exit Options," *MarketWatch*, June 19, 2013, accessed November 24, 2014, http://www .marketwatch.com/story/retirement-communities-read-the-contract-2013 -06-19.

26. Jane E. Zarem, ed., *Today's Continuing Care Retirement Community (CCRC)* (CRC Task Force, July 2010), 10–11, accessed October 20, 2014, https://www.seniorshousing.org/filephotos/research/CCRC_whitepaper .pdf; "Frequently Asked Questions," Newbridge on the Charles, accessed October 20, 2014, http://www.hebrewseniorlife.org/newbridge-frequently -asked-questions.

27. CARF-CCAC, *Consumer Guide to Understanding Financial Performance and Reporting in Continuing Care Retirement Communities* (Washington, DC: CARF-CCAC, 2007), 6, accessed October 20, 2014, http://www.carf.org/FinancialPerformanceCCRCs/; Abigail Jones, "Some Retirees Opting for Campus Life," *New York Times*, December 3, 2010, accessed October 20, 2014, http://newoldage.blogs.nytimes .com/2010/12/03/some-retirees-opting-for-campus-life/?_php=true& _type=blogs&_r=0.

28. Jane Gross, "Doctor Focuses on the Minds of the Elderly," *New York Times*, April 30, 2011, accessed October 20, 2014, http://www.nytimes.com/2011/05/01/us/01elderly.html?pagewanted=all.

29. Mary Ann Erickson et al., "Social Integration and the Move to a Continuing Care Retirement Community," in *Social Integration in the Second Half of Life*, ed. Karl Pillemer et al. (Baltimore, MD: Johns Hopkins University Press, 2000), 224. The average age of respondents was 76.5, and their ages ranged from 64 to 94. Approximately two-third were female, and two-thirds were married. Their median annual income was $75,000, and 60 percent had a graduate degree. Ibid., 217.

30. Kristi Rahrig Jenkins, Amy Mehraban Pienta, and Ann L. Horgas, "Activity and Health-Related Quality of Life in Continuing Care Retirement Communities," *Research on Aging* 24 (2002): 146.

31. Abir K. Bekhet, Jaclene A. Zauszniewski, and Wagdy E. Nakhla, "Reasons for Relocation to Retirement Communities: A Qualitative Study," *Western Journal of Nursing Research* 31, no. 4 (2009): 463–465; Lisa Groger and Jennifer Kinney, "CCRC Here We Come! Reasons for Moving to a Continuing Care Retirement Community," *Journal of Housing for the Elderly* 20, no. 4 (2006): 98–100.

32. "About Continuing Care Retirement Communities: What They Are and How They Work," AARP, accessed October 20, 2014, http://www.aarp.org/relationships/caregiving-resource-center/info-09-2010/ho_continuing_care_retirement_communities.html.

33. Paula Span, "Now, Tables for (Almost) Everyone," *New York Times*, March 6, 2012, accessed October 20, 2014, http://newoldage.blogs.nytimes.com/2012/03/06/now-tables-for-almost-everyone/.

34. Ashlea Ebeling, "Continuing Care Communities: A Big Investment with Catches," *Forbes*, September 26, 2011, accessed October 20, 2014, http://www.forbes.com/sites/ashleaebeling/2011/09/26/continuing-care-communities-a-big-investment-with-catches/.

35. Mather LifeWays Institute on Aging, Ziegler, and Brecht Associates, Inc., *Final Report of National Survey of Family Members of Residents Living in Continuing Care Retirement Communities* (2011), 18, accessed October 20, 2014, http://www.nxtbook.com/nxtbooks/mather/finalreport2011/#/18.

36. Ibid., 7; "About Continuing Care Retirement Communities," AARP; Ebeling, "Continuing Care Communities."

37. CARF-CCAC, *Consumer Guide to Understanding Financial Performance and Reporting in Continuing Care Retirement Communities*, 2.

38. "About Continuing Care Retirement Communities," AARP.

39. Ibid.; United States Senate Special Committee on Aging, *Continuing Care Retirement Communities: Risks to Seniors: Summary of Committee Investigation* (2010), 2, accessed October 20, 2014, http://riverwoodsrc.org/sites/default/files/PDFs/Senate_Report.pdf; CARF-CCAC, *Consumer Guide*

to *Understanding Financial Performance and Reporting in Continuing Care Retirement Communities*, 3–4; United States Government Accountability Office, *Older Americans: Continuing Care Retirement Communities Can Provide Benefits, but Not Without Some Risk* (2010), 5–6, accessed October 20, 2014, http://www.gao.gov/new.items/d10611.pdf.

40. CARF-CCAC, *Consumer Guide to Understanding Financial Performance and Reporting in Continuing Care Retirement Communities*, 5.

41. Ibid., 6.

42. Ibid.

43. Ebeling, "Continuing Care Communities."

44. United States Senate Special Committee on Aging, *Continuing Care Retirement Communities: Risks to Seniors*, 10–11 (discussing the 2009 bankruptcy filing by Erickson Retirement communities, one of the largest CCRC developers with 18 facilities serving 22,000 residents in multiple states); Elizabeth Olson, "Concerns Rise about Continuing-Care Enclaves," *New York Times*, September 15, 2010, accessed October 20, 2014, http://www.nytimes.com/2010/09/16/business/retirementspecial/16CARE.html?pagewanted=all&_r=0.

45. United States Government Accountability Office, *Older Americans: Continuing Care Retirement Communities Can Provide Benefits, but Not Without Some Risk*, 21–22; CARF-CCAC, *Consumer Guide to Understanding Financial Performance and Reporting in Continuing Care Retirement Communities*, 10.

46. See Nursing Home Reform Act, 42 U.S.C §1396r, 42 U.S.C. §1395i-3, 42 CFR §§483.15-483.75; "NH Regulations Plus: State Regulation by State," University of Minnesota Long-Term Care Resource Center, accessed October 20, 2014, http://www.hpm.umn.edu/nhregsplus/NHRegs_by_State/By%20State%20Main.html (last modified March 19, 2012); "Assisted Living Regulations and Licensing," Assisted Living Federation of America, accessed October 20, 2014, http://www.alfa.org/alfa/State_Regulations_and_Licensing_Informat.asp (detailing state regulations).

47. United States Senate Special Committee on Aging, *Continuing Care Retirement Communities: Risks to Seniors*, 1–2.

48. United States Government Accountability Office, *Older Americans: Continuing Care Retirement Communities Can Provide Benefits, but Not Without Some Risk*, 11–32.

49. "List of CARF-CCAC Accredited Continuing Care Retirement Communities (2014)," CARF International, accessed November 20, 2014, http://carf.org/ccrcListing.aspx.

50. Span, *When the Time Comes*, 132.

51. "Calaroga Terrace," ProviderData, accessed October 20, 2014, http://www.providerdata.com/portland-or/167258/calaroga-terrace.aspx.

52. Ebeling, "Continuing Care Communities."

53. Judith Graham, "A Choice of Community Care, in Your Own Home," *New York Times*, September 17, 2012, accessed October 20, 2014, http://newoldage.blogs.nytimes.com/2012/09/17/a-choice-of-community-care-but-in-your-own-home/.

54. United States Senate Special Committee on Aging, *Continuing Care Retirement Communities: Risks to Seniors*, 7.

55. "What to Ask and Observe When Visiting Continuing Care Retirement Communities," AARP, accessed October 20, 2014, http://www.aarp.org/relationships/caregiving-resource-center/info-09-2010/ho_what_to_ask_retirement_communities.html; CARF-CCAC, *Consumer Guide to Understanding Financial Performance and Reporting in Continuing Care Retirement Communities*, 12–14; California Advocates for Nursing Home Reform, *Points to Consider for CCRC Consumers* (San Francisco, CA: CANHR, 2009), accessed October 20, 2014, http://canhr.org/publications/PDFs/CCRCPtsToConsider.pdf.

CHAPTER 3

1. "DMMs and You," American Association of Daily Money Managers, accessed October 16, 2014, http://www.aadmm.com/dmms_and_you.htm.

2. Ibid.; Anne Tergesen, "A Little Help with the Bills," *Wall Street Journal*, July 27, 2012, accessed October 16, 2014, http://online.wsj.com/articles/SB10000872396390444840104577550910299244458.

3. "Search for AADMM Members," American Association of Daily Money Managers, accessed November 9, 2014, http://www.aadmm.com/findDMM.php.

4. Tergesen, "A Little Help with the Bills."

5. "Code of Ethics," American Association of Daily Money Managers, accessed October 16, 2014, http://www.aadmm.com/code_of_ethics.htm.

6. "ADMM's Certification Process—Frequently Asked Questions," American Association of Daily Money Managers, accessed October 16, 2014, http://www.aadmm.com/certification_faq.htm; "Eligibility and Application Process for Professional Daily Money Manager Certification," American Association of Daily Money Managers, accessed October 16, 2014, http://www.aadmm.com/certification/14/pdmm_candidate_requirements_2014.pdf. The minimum 1,500 hours of experience must include at least 1,250 of paid work and 250 of eligible pro bono work.

7. "List of Certified Professional Daily Money Managers," American Association of Daily Money Managers, accessed November 25, 2014, http://www.aadmm.com/certification_list.htm.

8. Tergesen, "A Little Help with the Bills."

9. Kathleen Michon, "Daily Money Management Programs for Seniors," *Nolo*, accessed October 16, 2014, http://www.nolo.com/legal-encyclopedia/daily-money-management-programs-seniors-32269.html.

10. Cathy Jo Cress, *Handbook of Geriatric Care Management*, 3rd ed. (Burlington, MA: Jones & Bartlett Learning, 2012), 3.

11. "What You Need to Know," National Association of Professional Geriatric Care Managers, accessed October 16, 2014, http://www.caremanager.org /why-care-management/what-you-should-know/.

12. Lisa M. Scott and Candace Sharkey, "Putting the Pieces Together: Private-Duty Home Healthcare and Geriatric Care Management: One Home Health Agency's Model," *Home Healthcare Nurse* 25, no. 3 (2007): 168.

13. "What You Need to Know," National Association of Professional Geriatric Care Managers.

14. Scott and Sharkey, "Private-Duty Home Healthcare and Geriatric Care Management," 168.

15. Ibid.

16. "Find a Care Manager," National Association of Professional Geriatric Care Managers, accessed October 16, 2014, http://memberfinder .caremanager.org/.

17. Caring.com Staff, "Geriatric Care Managers," accessed October 16, 2014, http://www.caring.com/local/geriatric-care-managers.

18. Marilyn Wideman, "Geriatric Care Management: Role, Need, and Benefits," *Home Healthcare Nurse* 30, no. 9 (2012): 556.

19. Susan M. Enguidanos and Paula M. Jamison, "Moving from Tacit Knowledge to Evidence-Based Practice: The Kaiser Permanente Community Partners Study," *Home Health Care Service Quarterly* 25, no. 1–2 (2006): 27.

20. Robert Abrams, "Are You a Planner or a Gambler?," *New York State Bar Association Journal* (July–August 2011): 6–7.

21. "What Is an Elder Law Attorney?," Area Agency on Aging, accessed October 16, 2014, http://www.agingcarefl.org/aging/legal; Rebecca C. Morgan, "The Future of Elder Law Practice," *William Mitchell Law Review* 37, no. 1 (2010): 21.

22. "NAELA's History," National Academy of Elder Law Attorneys, accessed November 25, 2014, http://www.naela.org/Public/About /Fact_Sheet/NAELA_s_History/Public/About_NAELA/History .aspx?hkey=8b2aab86-18e9-48cb-af8d-6afadee9f0f4; Timothy L. Takacs, "The Life Care Plan: Integrating a Healthcare-Focused Approach to Meeting the Needs of Your Clients and Families into Your Elder Law Practice," *NAELA Quarterly* 16 (2003): 4–6; Paula P. Tchirkow, "Advocates for the Elderly and 'Eyes and Ears' for Elder Law Attorneys," *Pennsylvania Lawyer* 24 (2002): 35.

23. Morgan, "The Future of Elder Law Practice," 12.

24. National Academy of Elder Law Attorneys, accessed October 16, 2014, http://www.naela.org/.

25. "Find a CELA," National Elder Law Foundation, accessed November 9, 2014, http://www.nelf.org/find-a-cela.

26. "About NELF," National Elder Law Foundation, accessed December 2, 2014, http://www.nelf.org/about-nelf.

27. Harry Wang, "Tech Advances Will Give Aging Baby Boomers More Independence," *E-Commerce Times*, October 1, 2014, accessed December 2, 2014, http://www.ecommercetimes.com/story/81128.html.

28. Virginia Hessels, Glenn S. Le Prell, and William C. Mann, "Advances in Personal Emergency Response and Detection Systems," *Assistive Technology* 23, no. 3 (2011): 155; Kristen De San Miguel and Gill Lewin, "Personal Emergency Alarms: What Impact Do They Have on Older People's Lives?," *Australasian Journal on Ageing* 27, no. 2 (2008): 103–105.

29. "Our Profession," National Association of Professional Organizers, accessed October 16, 2014, http://www.napo.net/our_profession/.

30. Cantheclutter, accessed October 16, 2014, http://cantheclutter.com/.

31. "The Basics of Home Staging," Define by Redesign, accessed October 16, 2014, http://www.definebyredesign.com/services/homestaging.php.

32. Debra Sacks et al., "The Value of Daily Money Management: An Analysis of Outcomes and Costs," *Journal of Evidence-Based Social Work* 9, no. 5 (2012): 507–508.

33. Ibid., 509–510.

34. Lisa Nerenberg, *Daily Money Management Programs: A Protection against Elder Abuse* (Washington, DC: National Center on Elder Abuse, 2003), accessed October 16, 2014, http://www.ncea.aoa.gov/Resources/Publication/docs/DailyMoneyManagement.pdf.

CHAPTER 4

1. Board of Governors of the Federal Reserve, *Insights into the Financial Experiences of Older Adults: A Forum Briefing Paper* (Washington, DC: Board of Governors of the Federal Reserve System, 2013), 21, accessed November 12, 2014, http://www.federalreserve.gov/newsevents/conferences/older-adults-forum-paper-20130717.pdf.

2. "2012 Alzheimer's Disease Facts and Figures," Alzheimer's Association, 14, accessed October 20, 2014, http://www.alz.org/downloads/facts_figures_2012.pdf.

3. Lawrence A. Frolik and Linda S. Whitton, *Everyday Law for Seniors* (Boulder, CO: Paradigm Publishers, 2012), 138–153.

4. American Bar Association Commission on Law and Aging, "Default Surrogate Consent Statutes" (June 2014), accessed March 19, 2015, http://www.americanbar.org/content/dam/aba/administrative/law_aging/2014_default_surrogate_consent_statutes.authcheckdam.pdf.

5. American Hospital Association, *Put It in Writing: Questions and Answers on Advance Directives* (American Hospital Association, 2012), 3, accessed October 20, 2014, http://www.aha.org/content/13/putitinwriting.pdf.

6. Diana Anderson, "Review of Advance Health Care Directive Laws in the United States, the Portability of Documents, and the Surrogate Decision Maker When No Document Is Executed," *National Academy of Elder Law Attorneys Journal* 8, no. 2 (2012): 186.

7. Ohio Revised Code §1337.17; Consolidated Laws of New York §2983.

8. Maria J. Silveira, Scott Y.H. Kim, and Kenneth M. Langa, "Advance Directives and Outcomes of Surrogate Decision Making before Death," *New England Journal of Medicine* 362 (2010): 1216.

9. Anderson, "Review of Advance Health Care Directive Laws in the United States," 183.

10. American Hospital Association, *Put It in Writing*, 4; Anderson, "Review of Advance Health Care Directive Laws in the United States," 190.

11. 42 U.S.C. §1395cc(f) (2010).

12. U.S. Department of Health and Human Services, Office of the Assistant Secretary for Planning and Evaluation (ASPE), *Advance Directives and Advance Care Planning: Report to Congress* (Washington, DC: ASPE, August 2008), x, accessed October 20, 2014, http://aspe.hhs.gov/daltcp/reports/2008/ADCongRpt.pdf.

13. Ibid., xi.

14. Deborah L. Jacobs, "How to Do Estate Planning on the Cheap," *Forbes*, November 19, 2010, accessed October 20, 2014, http://www.forbes.com/forbes/2010/1206/investment-guide-living-will-software-cheap-estate-planning.html.

15. Patrick Triplett et al., "Content of Advance Directives for Individuals with Advanced Dementia," *Journal of Aging and Health* 20, no. 5 (2008): 588; Susan P. Shapiro, "Advance Directives: The Elusive Goal of Having the Last Word," *Journal of the National Academy of Elder Law Attorneys* 8, no. 2 (2012): 218–219.

16. Patricia A. King, Lawrence O. Gostin, and Judith C. Areen, *Law, Medicine and Ethics* (New York: Foundation Press, 2006), 466.

17. Anderson, "Review of Advance Health Care Directive Laws in the United States," 187.

18. "State of Ohio Living Will Declaration," Cleveland Clinic, 3–4, accessed October 20, 2014, http://my.clevelandclinic.org/ccf/media/Files/Patients/OhioLivingWill.pdf.

19. Anderson, "Review of Advance Health Care Directive Laws in the United States," 186.

20. "State of Ohio Health Care Power of Attorney," Cleveland Clinic, 4–6, accessed October 20, 2014, http://my.clevelandclinic.org/Documents/Patients/health-care-power-of-attorney-form.pdf.

21. Benjamin H. Levi and Michael J. Green, "Too Soon to Give Up: Re-Examining the Value of Advance Directives," *American Journal of Bioethics* 10, no. 4 (2010): 18. Available at http://www.tandfonline.com/doi/pdf/10.1080/15265161003599691.

22. American Bar Association Commission on Law and Aging, *Consumer's Tool Kit for Health Care Advance Planning*, 2nd ed. (Washington, DC: American Bar Association on Law and Aging, 2005), Tool 1/page 1, accessed October 20, 2014, http://apps.americanbar.org/aging/publications/docs/consumer_tool_kit_bk.pdf.

23. Ibid.

24. Frolik and Whitton, *Everyday Law for Seniors*, 159.

25. "Donate the Gift of Life," U.S. Department of Health and Human Services, accessed October 20, 2014, http://www.organdonor.gov/index.html.

26. See California Probate Code §4701, Part 3.

27. "State of Ohio Living Will Declaration," 4.

28. "Advanced Directive Declaration for Mental Health Treatment," Behavioral Connections, accessed October 20, 2014, http://www.behavioralconnections.org/poc/view_doc.php?type=doc&id=8992; "What You Should Know about the Declaration of Mental Health Treatment," Ohio State Bar Association, accessed October 20, 2014, https://www.ohiobar.org/ForPublic/Resources/LawYouCanUse/Pages/LawYouCanUse-298.aspx.

29. "Do All States Specifically Have PAD Statutes?," National Resource Center on Psychiatric Advance Directives, accessed October 20, 2014, http://www.nrc-pad.org/faqs/do-all-states-specifically-have-pad-statutes.

30. Lisa Brodoff, "Planning for Alzheimer's Disease with Mental Health Advance Directives," *The Elder Law Journal* 17, no. 2 (2010): 256.

31. Ibid.

32. Ibid.

33. Ohio Revised Code 2135.07(B).

34. Sabatino, "10 Legal Myths About Advance Medical Directives," 2.

35. ASPE, *Advance Directives and Advance Care Planning*, xi.

36. Shapiro, "The Elusive Goal of Having the Last Word," 216.

37. Levi and Green, "Re-Examining the Value of Advance Directives," 18.

38. Shapiro, "The Elusive Goal of Having the Last Word," 220.

39. Ibid., 221–222.

40. Michael J. Newton, "Precedent Autonomy: Life-Sustaining Intervention and the Demented Patient," *Cambridge Quarterly of Healthcare Ethics* 8, no. 2 (1999): 190.

41. Stephen G. Post, "Alzheimer Disease and the 'Then' Self," *Kennedy Institute of Ethics Journal* 5, no. 4 (1995): 317–318.

42. Rebecca Dresser, "Dworkin on Dementia: Elegant Theory, Questionable Policy," *Hastings Center Report* 25, no. 6 (1995): 33; Rebecca Dresser, "Missing Persons: Legal Perceptions of Incompetent Patients," *Rutgers Law Review* 46, no. 2 (1994): 718–719.

43. Ronald Dworkin, *Life's Dominion: An Argument about Abortion, Euthanasia, and Individual Freedom* (New York: Vintage, 1994), 222–229; Newton, "Precedent Autonomy," 192–193.

44. Sara T. Fry et al., "Evolution of a Home Health Ethics Committee," *Home Healthcare Nurse* 19, no. 9 (2001): 565–566.

45. Mark P. Aulisio and Robert M. Arnold, "Role of the Ethics Committee: Helping to Address Value Conflicts or Uncertainties," *Chest* 134, no. 2 (2008): 418–422.

46. Frolik and Whitton, *Everyday Law for Seniors*, 160–161.

47. Eric Widera et al., "Finances in the Older Patient With Cognitive Impairment: 'He Didn't Want Me to Take Over'," *Journal of the American Medical Association* 305, no. 7 (2011): 705.

48. Ibid., 701.

49. "Wills and Probate: Financial Power of Attorney," Ohio Legal Services, accessed October 20, 2014, http://www.ohiolegalservices.org /public/legal_problem/wills-and-probate/financial-power-of-attorney /qandact_view; Steve Weisman, *A Guide to Elder Planning: Everything You Need to Know to Protect Your Loved Ones and Yourself* (Upper Saddle River, NJ: FT Press, 2013), 27.

50. Walecia Konrad, "Old, Infirm and at the Center of a Legal Struggle," *New York Times*, November 13, 2012, accessed October 20, 2014, http://www .nytimes.com/2012/11/14/your-money/old-infirm-and-in-the-center-of-a -lawsuit.html?gwh=421D6CFD2852591EF9998620ABDDC488&gwt =pay.

51. Frolik and Whitton, *Everyday Law for Seniors*, 162–163.

52. "Power of Attorney," Uniform Law Commission, accessed October 20, 2014, http://www.uniformlaws.org/Act.aspx?title=Power%20of%20Attorney.

53. Ibid.; Charles P. Sabatino, "Damage Prevention and Control for Financial Incapacity," *Journal of the American Medical Association* 305, no.7 (2011): 708.

54. Konrad, "Old, Infirm and at the Center of a Legal Struggle" Sandra Block, "Power of Attorney Can be Valuable and Dangerous Tool," *USA Today*, December 8, 2008, accessed October 20, 2014, http://usatoday30.usatoday .com/money/perfi/columnist/block/2008-12-08-managing-money -power-attorney_N.htm?csp=N009.

55. See *Statute of Descent and Distribution*, Ohio Revised Code §2105.06 (2012).

56. Jacobs, "How to Do Estate Planning on the Cheap."

57. Frolik and Whitton, *Everyday Law for Seniors*, 163–165.

58. "Transfer on Death (TOD) Registration," U.S. Securities and Exchange Commission, accessed October 20, 2014, http://www.sec.gov/answers /todreg.htm.

59. "Funeral Costs and Pricing Checklist," Federal Trade Commission, accessed October 20, 2014, http://www.consumer.ftc.gov/articles /0301-funeral-costs-and-pricing-checklist#Calculating.

60. *Consumer's Tool Kit for Health Care Advance Planning*, American Bar Association Commission on Law and Aging, accessed December 1, 2014, http://www.americanbar.org/groups/law_aging/resources/health_care _decision_making/consumer_s_toolkit_for_health_care_advance _planning.html.

61. *Consumer's Tool Kit for Health Care Advance Planning*, Tool 8.

62. Maryland State Advisory Council on Quality Care at the End of Life, *Study on a Statewide Advance Directive Registry* (2005), ii, accessed October 20, 2014, http://www.oag.state.md.us/Healthpol/ADregistry .pdf; Patrice Eller and Peter Tommasulo, *Advance Directive Registries: A Policy Opportunity* (Center for Healthcare Research and Transformation, 2011), accessed October 20, 2014, http://www.chrt.org/public-policy /policy-papers/advance-directive-registries-a-policy-opportunity/.

63. "Advance Directive Notification," American Hospital Association, accessed October 20, 2014, http://www.aha.org/content/13/piiw-walletcard .pdf.

64. "Frequently Asked Questions (FAQ) about the U.S. Living Will Registry," U.S. Living Will Registry, accessed October 20, 2014, http://www .uslivingwillregistry.com/faq.shtm.

65. Silveira et al., "Advance Directives and Outcomes of Surrogate Decision Making before Death," 1218.

CHAPTER 5

1. Mark Gillispie, "Driver in Fatal Hit-Skip Avoids Prison Time," *Cleveland Plain Dealer*, January 15, 2013, B3.

2. Michael Winter, "100-Year-Old Driver Injures 9 Kids, 2 Adults Near School," *USA Today*, August 29, 2012, accessed October 21, 2014, http://content.usatoday.com/communities/ondeadline/post/2012/08 /driver-101-hits-parents-kids-outside-la-school-8-hurt/1.

3. Joel Rubin, Daren Briscoe, and Mitchell Landsberg, "Car Plows Through Crowd in Santa Monica, Killing 9," *Los Angeles Times*, July 17, 2003, accessed October 21, 2014, http://articles.latimes.com/2003/jul/17/local /me-smcrash17.

4. Nicole Kaplan and Monika White, for the Center for Healthy Aging, *Getting Around: Alternatives for Seniors Who No Longer Drive* (Washington, DC: AAA Foundation for Traffic Safety, 2007), 12–19, accessed October 21, 2014, https://www.aaafoundation.org/sites/default/files /GettingAroundReport.pdf.

5. Kevin DeGood et al., *Aging in Place, Stuck without Options: Fixing the Mobility Crisis Threatening the Baby Boom Generation*. Transportation for America, 2011, 4, accessed October 21, 2014, http://t4america.org/docs /SeniorsMobilityCrisis.pdf.

6. Federal Highway Administration, "Distribution of Licensed Drivers—2012: By Sex and Percentage in Each Age Group and Relation to Population Table DL-20," in Office of Highway Policy Information, *Highway Statistics 2012* (Washington, DC: Federal Highway Administration, 2014), DL-20, accessed November 25, 2014, http://www.fhwa.dot.gov /policyinformation/statistics/2012/index.cfm.

7. Shelley Emling, "Study Shows Surprising Number of Drivers Over 100," *The Huffington Post*, September 23, 2013, accessed October 21, 2014, http://www.huffingtonpost.com/2013/09/23/older-drivers_n_3975579 .html.

8. National Highway Traffic Safety Administration, *Traffic Safety Facts 2012: A Compilation of Motor Vehicle Crash Data from the Fatality Analysis Reporting System and the General Estimates System*, DOT HS 812 032 (Washington, DC: National Highway Traffic Safety Administration, 2014), 28, accessed November 26, 2014, http://www-nrd.nhtsa.dot .gov/Pubs/812032.pdf.

9. "Older Adult Drivers: Get the Facts," Centers for Disease Control and Prevention, accessed October 21, 2014, http://www.cdc.gov /Motorvehiclesafety/Older_Adult_Drivers/adult-drivers_factsheet.html; Brian Tefft, "Risks Older Drivers Pose to Themselves and to Other Road Users," *Journal of Safety Research* 39, no. 6 (2008): 580–581.

10. "Older Adult Drivers: Get the Facts," Centers for Disease Control and Prevention.

11. E. Braver and R. Trempel, "Are Older Drivers Actually at Higher Risk of Involvement in Collisions Resulting in Deaths or Non-fatal Injuries among Their Passengers and Other Road Users?," *Injury Prevention* 10, no. 1 (2004): 30–31.

12. Ivan Cheung and Anne T. McCartt, "Declines in Fatal Crashes of Older Drivers: Changes in Crash Risk and Survivability," *Accident Analysis and Prevention* 43, no. 3 (2011): 669; National Highway Traffic Safety Administration, *Traffic Safety Facts 2012*, 200.

13. Braver, "Are Older Drivers Actually at Higher Risk of Involvement in Collisions Resulting in Deaths or Non-fatal Injuries among Their Passengers and Other Road Users?," 30–31; John Eberhard, "Older Drivers' 'High Per-Mile Crash Involvement': The Implications for Licensing Authorities," *Traffic Injury Prevention* 9, no. 4 (2008): 287; Highway Loss Data Institute, "Estimating the Effect of Projected Changes in the Driving Population on Collision Claim Frequency," *Highway Loss Data Institute Bulletin* 29, no. 8 (2012), 6–8, accessed October 21, 2014, http://www.iihs .org/research/topics/pdf/HLDI_bulletin_29.8.pdf.

14. "Older Drivers: November 2014," Insurance Institute for Highway Safety, accessed November 12, 2014, http://www.iihs.org/iihs/topics/laws /olderdrivers.

15. *California's Three-Tier Driving-Centered Assessment System*: *Outcome Analysis*, State of California Department of Motor Vehicles, 2011, vi, accessed October 21, 2014, http://apps.dmv.ca.gov/about/profile/rd/r_d _report/Section_2/S2-234.pdf.

16. Karlene K. Ball et al., "Can High-Risk Older Drivers Be Identified Through Performance-Based Measures in a Department of Motor Vehicles Setting?," *Journal of the American Geriatrics Society* 54, no. 1 (2006): 81.

17. American Medical Association and National Highway Traffic Safety Association, *Physician's Guide to Assessing and Counseling Older Drivers*, 2nd ed. (Chicago, IL: American Medical Association, 2010), 43–44, accessed November 4, 2014, http://www.aarp.org/content/dam/aarp /livable-communities/plan/transportation/older-drivers-guide.pdf.

18. Ediriweera Desapriya et al., "Vision Screening of Older Drivers for Preventing Road Traffic Injuries and Fatalities," *Cochrane Database of Systematic Reviews* 2 (2014): CD006252; David C. Grabowski, Christine M. Campbell, and Michael A. Morrisey, "Elderly Licensure Laws and Motor Vehicle Fatalities," *Journal of the American Medical Association* 291, no. 23 (2004): 2840; Jim Langford et al., "Some Consequences of Different Older Driver Licensing Procedures in Australia," *Accident Analysis & Prevention* 36, no. 6 (2004): 998–1000.

19. Elena Kulikov, "The Social and Policy Predictors of Driving Mobility among Older Adults," *Journal of Aging & Social Policy* 23, no. 1 (2011): 14.

20. "Q&A: Older Drivers," Insurance Institute for Highway Safety, March 2014, accessed November 26, 2014, http://www.iihs.org/iihs/topics/t/older -drivers/qanda; Cynthia Owsley et al., "Impact of an Educational Program on the Safety of High-Risk, Visually Impaired, Older Drivers," *American Journal of Preventive Medicine* 26, no. 3 (2004): 225–28; Glenyth E. Nasvadi and John Vavrik, "Crash Risk of Older Drivers after Attending a Mature Driver Education Program," *Accident Analysis & Prevention* 39, no. 6 (2007): 1079.

21. "Physician Reporting of At-Risk Drivers," AAA Foundation for Traffic Safety, accessed October 21, 2014, http://lpp.seniordrivers.org/lpp/index .cfm?selection=reportingdrs1&orderby=abbv&sortorder=asc&country= USA; American Medical Association and National Highway Traffic Safety Association, *Physician's Guide to Assessing and Counseling Older Drivers*. The states are California, Delaware, Georgia, Maine, New Jersey, Nevada, Oregon, and Pennsylvania.

22. "Family & Friend Reporting of At-Risk Drivers," AAA Foundation for Traffic Safety, accessed October 21, 2014, http://lpp.seniordrivers.org/lpp/ index.cfm?selection=reportingfamilyfriends1; "How Family/Friends Report," AAA Foundation for Traffic Safety, accessed October 21, 2014, http://lpp .seniordrivers.org/lpp/index.cfm?selection=reportingfamilyfriends2.

23. "Law Enforcement Reporting of At-Risk Drivers," AAA Foundation for Traffic Safety, accessed October 21, 2014, http://lpp.seniordrivers.org/lpp/index.cfm?selection=lawenforcement.

24. "Driver Medical Review Process / States WITH Medical Advisory Board (MAB)," AAA Foundation for Traffic Safety, accessed October 21, 2014, http://lpp.seniordrivers.org/lpp/index.cfm?selection=statesMAB; "Driver Medical Review Process / States WITHOUT Medical Advisory Board (MAB)," AAA Foundation for Traffic Safety, accessed October 21, 2014, http://lpp.seniordrivers.org/lpp/index.cfm?selection=statesnoMAB; "Types of Conditions or Restrictions on Licenses, Page 1," AAA Foundation for Traffic Safety, accessed October 21, 2014, http://lpp.seniordrivers.org/lpp/index.cfm?selection=restrictedlicensetypes1.

25. Kulikov, "The Social and Policy Predictors of Driving Mobility among Older Adults."

26. "Older Adult Drivers: Get the Facts," Centers for Disease Control and Prevention.

27. "Q&A: Older Drivers," Insurance Institute for Highway Safety.

28. Lorraine Sommerfeld, "Drive, She Said: New Test Coming Soon for Elderly Ontario Drivers," *The Globe and Mail*, January 31, 2014, accessed October 21, 2014, http://www.theglobeandmail.com/globe-drive/news/new-test-coming-soon-for-elderly-ontario-drivers/article16638607/.

29. "We Need to Talk: Family Conversation with Older Drivers, Module 2," AARP, accessed October 21, 2014, http://www.aarp.org/home-garden/transportation/we_need_to_talk/?cmp=RDRCT-WNTT.

30. Ibid.

31. Chandra C. Goreman et al., *Senior Transportation Alternatives: Why Are They Important and What Makes Them Work?* (Tampa, FL: NCTR at CUTR, 2003), accessed October 21, 2014, http://www.nctr.usf.edu/pdf/473-09.pdf.

32. Nina Glasgow, "An Intervention to Improve Transportation Arrangements," in *Social Integration in the Second Half of Life*, ed. Karl Pillemer et al. (Baltimore, MD: Johns Hopkins University Press, 2000), 244–245.

33. Sven A. Beiker, "Legal Aspects of Autonomous Driving," *Santa Clara Law Review* 52, no. 4 (2012): 1147–1148.

34. "Smart Features for Older Drivers," AAA Association Communication, 6, accessed October 21, 2014, http://seniordriving.aaa.com/sites/default/files/Smart-Features-for-Older-Drivers-Brochure.pdf.

35. James W. Jenness et al., *Use of Advanced In-Vehicle Technology by Young and Older Early Adopters: Survey Results on Adaptive Cruise Control Systems* (March 2008), Report No. DOT HS 810 917 (Washington, DC: National Highway Traffic Safety Administration, 2008), 1–3.

36. John Markoff and Somini Sengupta, "Drivers with Hands Full Get a Backup: The Car," *New York Times*, January 12, 2013, accessed October

21, 2014, http://www.nytimes.com/2013/01/12/science/drivers-with-hands-full-get-a-backup-the-car.html?pagewanted=all.

37. "2014 Mercedes-Benz E-Class Introduces 'Intelligent Drive'," *J.D. Power*, December 17, 2012, accessed October 21, 2014, http://autos.jdpower.com/content/blog-post/apv6Qyy/2014-mercedes-benz-e-class-introduces-intelligent-drive.htm.

38. Beiker, "Legal Aspects of Autonomous Driving," 1148.

39. Nidhi Karla, James Anderson, and Martin Wachs, *Liability and Regulation of Autonomous Vehicle Technologies: California PATH Research Report UCB-ITS-PRR-2009-28* (Arlington, VA: RAND, 2009), 17–36, accessed October 21, 2014, http://www.dot.ca.gov/newtech/researchreports/reports/2009/prr-2009-28_liability_reg_&_auto_vehicle_final_report_2009.pdf; John Markoff, "Collision in the Making between Self-Driving Cars and How the World Works," *New York Times*, January 23, 2011, accessed October 21, 2014, http://www.nytimes.com/2012/01/24/technology/googles-autonomous-vehicles-draw-skepticism-at-legal-symposium.html?_r=0; Tom Vanderbilt, "Let the Robot Drive: The Autonomous Car of the Future Is Here," *Wired Magazine*, January 20, 2012, accessed October 21, 2014, http://www.wired.com/magazine/2012/01/ff_autonomouscars; KPMG, *Self-Driving Cars: The Next Revolution* (KPMG and Center for Automotive Research, 2012), 19–22, accessed October 21, 2014, https://www.kpmg.com/US/en/IssuesAndInsights/ArticlesPublications/Documents/self-driving-cars-next-revolution.pdf.

CHAPTER 6

1. Richard Russo, *Elsewhere: A Memoir* (New York: Knopf, 2012), 167 and 181.

2. Tracy Weber, Charles Ornstein, and Jennifer LaFleur, "Dangers Found in Lack of Safety Oversight for Medicare Drug Benefit," *Washington Post*, May 11, 2013, accessed October 20, 2014, http://www.washingtonpost.com/national/health-science/dangers-found-in-lack-of-safety-oversight-for-medicare-drug-benefit/2013/05/11/067a10ae-b8ec-11e2-aa9e-a02b765ff0ea_story.html.

3. Centers for Disease Control and Prevention, "Therapeutic Drug Use," *FastStats*, accessed November 20, 2014, http://www.cdc.gov/nchs/fastats/drug-use-therapeutic.htm (citing United States Department of Health and Human Services, *Health, United States, 2013 with Special Feature on Prescription Drugs* [Hyattsville, MD: 2014], table 92, accessed November 20, 2014 http://www.cdc.gov/nchs/data/hus/hus13.pdf).

4. Wenjun Zhong et al., "Age and Sex Patterns of Drug Prescribing in a Defined American Population," *Mayo Clinic Proceedings* 88, no. 7 (2013): 704.

5. Shannon Brownlee, *Overtreated: Why Too Much Medicine Is Making Us Sicker and Poorer* (New York: Bloomsbury, 2007), 183.

6. Gregg A. Warshaw, Elizabeth J. Bragg, and Ruth W. Shaull, *Geriatric Medicine Training and Practice in the United States at the Beginning of the 21st Century* (The Association of Directors of Geriatric Academic Programs, July 2002), 25, accessed October 20, 2014, http://www.americangeriatrics .org/files/documents/gwps/ADGAP%20Full%20Report.pdf.

7. Ibid.; "Geriatrics Basic Facts & Information," Healthinaging.org, accessed October 20, 2014, http://www.healthinaging.org/aging-and-health-a-to-z /topic:geriatrics/.

8. Ken Duckworth, *Depression in Older Persons Fact Sheet* (National Alliance on Mental Illness, 2009), 1, accessed October 20, 2014, http://www .nami.org/Content/NavigationMenu/Mental_Illnesses/Depression/Depres- sion_Older_Persons_FactSheet_2009.pdf.

9. Elizabeth J. Bragg et al., "The Development of Academic Geriatric Medicine in the United States 2005 to 2010: An Essential Resource for Improving the Medical Care of Older Adults," *Journal of the American Geriatrics Society* 60, no. 8 (2012): 1543.

10. Barbara Starfield et al., "Ambulatory Specialist Use by Nonhospitalized Patients in US Health Plans: Correlates and Consequences," *Journal of Ambulatory Care Management* 32, no. 3 (2009): 218, 222.

11. Joseph Pergolizzi et al., "Opioids and the Management of Chronic Severe Pain in the Elderly: Consensus Statement of an International Expert Panel with Focus on the Six Clinically Most Often Used World Health Organization Step III Opioids (Buprenorphine, Fentanyl, Hydromor- phone, Methadone, Morphine, Oxycodone)," *Pain Practice* 8, no. 4 (2008): 290.

12. Alyssa Brown, "Chronic Pain Rates Shoot Up Until Americans Reach Late 50s," *Gallup Wellbeing*, April 27, 2012, accessed October 20, 2014, http:// www.gallup.com/poll/154169/chronic-pain-rates-shoot-until-americans -reach-late-50s.aspx.

13. Atul Gawande, "The Way We Age Now," *New Yorker*, April 30, 2007, accessed October 20, 2014, http://www.newyorker.com/magazine/2007/04/30 /the-way-we-age-now.

14. Ibid.

15. Ibid.

16. "FAQ's," American Geriatrics Society, accessed October 20, 2014, http:// www.americangeriatrics.org/advocacy_public_policy/gwps/gwps_faqs /id:3183.

17. Bragg et al., "The Development of Academic Geriatric Medicine in the United States 2005 to 2010," 1540; John Y. Campbell et al., "The Unknown Profession: A Geriatrician," *Journal of the American Geriatrics Society* 61, no. 3 (2013): 447.

18. *Statement of John W. Rowe Before the Special Committee on Aging, U.S. Senate* (April 16, 2008), 4, accessed October 21, 2014, http://www.iom.edu /~/media/Files/Report%20Files/2008/Retooling-for-an-Aging-America -Building-the-Health-Care-Workforce/Statement%20of%20John%20W%20 Rowe%20MD%20Before%20the%20Special%20Committee%20on%20 Aging%20US%20Senate%20April%2016%202008.pdf.

19. Ibid.; Dilip V. Jeste, "Aging and Mental Health: Bad News and Good News," *Psychiatric News* (from the American Psychiatric Association), July 6, 2012, accessed November 6, 2014, http://psychnews.psychiatryonline .org/doi/full/10.1176/pn.47.13.psychnews_47_13_3-a.

20. Institute for Oral Health 2008 Focus Group #1 on "Oral Health in Aging America," *Oral Health Needs for Seniors: Challenges and Solutions in Dental Care for Aging Adults* (Institute for Oral Health, 2008), 7, accessed October 21, 2014, http://iohwa.org/2008fg/IOHFeb08FocusGroup_whitepaper.pdf.

21. Lars E. Peterson et al., "Rural-Urban Distribution of the U.S. Geriatrics Physician Workforce," *Journal of the American Geriatrics Society* 59, no. 4 (2011): 700–702.

22. Bragg et al., "The Development of Academic Geriatric Medicine in the United States 2005 to 2010," 1540.

23. Campbell et al., "The Unknown Profession: A Geriatrician," 447.

24. Center for Workforce Studies Association of American Medical Colleges, *Recent Studies and Reports on Physician Shortages in the US* (AAMC, 2012), 14, accessed October 21, 2014, https://www.aamc.org /download/100598/data/recentworkforcestudies.pdf.

25. Ibid.

26. Bragg et al., "The Development of Academic Geriatric Medicine in the United States 2005 to 2010," 1542, 1544.

27. Ibid., 1544.

28. Barbara Starfield et al., "Comorbidity and the Use of Primary Care and Specialist Care in the Elderly," *Annals of Family Medicine* 3, no. 3 (2005): 220.

29. Marsha Mercer, "How to Beat the Doctor Shortage," *AARP Bulletin*, March 2013, accessed October 21, 2014, http://www.aarp.org/health /medicare-insurance/info-03-2013/how-to-beat-doctor-shortage.html.

30. Bernard Sanders, Subcommittee on Primary Health and Aging, U.S. Senate Committee on Health, Education, Labor & Pensions, *Primary Care Access: 30 Million New Patients and 11 Months to Go: Who Will Provide Their Primary Care?* (United States Senate, 2013), 1, accessed October 21, 2014, http:// www.sanders.senate.gov/imo/media/doc/PrimaryCareAccessReport.pdf.

31. Ibid.

32. Gawande, "The Way We Age Now."

33. Sharona Hoffman and Andy Podgurski, "E-Health Hazards: Provider Liability and Electronic Health Record Systems," *Berkeley Technology Law Journal* 24, no. 4 (2010): 1537–1555.

34. Michael T. French et al., "Is the United States Ready to Embrace Concierge Medicine?," *Population Health Management* 13, no. 4 (2010): 177; Nissa Simon, "Is a 'Boutique' Doctor for You? Here's What You Need to Know Before Signing Up with a 'Concierge' Practice," *AARP Health*, January 7, 2013, accessed October 21, 2014, http://www.aarp.org/health/healthy-living/info-01-2013/boutique-doctors.html.

35. Simon, "Is a 'Boutique' Doctor for You?"

36. C. J. Miles, "Concierge Medicine: An Alternative to Insurance," *Association of Mature American Citizens Health & Wealth*, June 26, 2014, accessed November 6, 2014, http://amac.us/concierge-medicine-alternative-insurance/.

37. French et al., "Is the United States Ready to Embrace Concierge Medicine?," 180–181; Peter A. Clark et al., "Concierge Medicine: Medical, Legal and Ethical Perspectives," *Internet Journal of Law, Healthcare and Ethics* 7, no. 1 (2011): 7; Stephen M. Petterson et al., "Projecting US Primary Care Physician Workforce Needs: 2010–2025," *Annals of Family Medicine* 10, no. 6 (2012): 505; Elizabeth O'Brien, "Why Concierge Medicine Will Get Bigger: Practices Could Shield Patients from Health-Care Turmoil," *MarketWatch* January 17, 2013, accessed October 21, 2014, http://www.aarp.org/health/healthy-living/info-01-2013/boutique-doctors.html.

38. Andrew Gottschalk and Susan A. Flocke, "Time Spent in Face-to-Face Patient Care and Work Outside the Examination Room," *Annals of Family Medicine* 3, no. 6 (2005): 491 (finding that the average time per patient was 13.3 minutes); Kimberly S. H. Yarnall et al., "Family Physicians as Team Leaders: 'Time' to Share the Care," *Preventing Chronic Disease: Public Health Research, Practice, and Policy* 6, no. 2 (2009): A59, accessed October 21, 2014, http://www.cdc.gov/pcd/issues/2009/apr/08_0023.htm (finding that the mean length for an acute care visit is 17.3 minutes, the mean for a chronic disease care visit is 19.3 minutes, and the average for a preventive care visit is 21.4 minutes, and that of total clinical time spent by physicians, these comprise 45.8 percent, 37.4 percent, and 16.8 percent, respectively); Kevin Fiscella and Ronald M. Epstein, "So Much to Do, So Little Time: Care for the Socially Disadvantaged and the 15-Minute Visit," *Archives of Internal Medicine* 168, no. 17 (2008): 1843 ("The average office visit in the United States lasts for about 16 minutes.").

39. Leana Wen and Joshua Kosowsky, *When Doctors Don't Listen: How to Avoid Misdiagnoses and Unnecessary Tests* (New York: St. Martin's Press, 2012), 196–198.

40. Ibid., 275.

41. Emily Oshima Lee and Ezekiel J. Emanuel, "Shared Decision Making to Improve Care and Reduce Costs," *New England Journal of Medicine* 368 (2013): 6–8.

42. Ibid.

43. Timothy J. Judson, Allan S. Detsky, and Matthew J. Press, "Encouraging Patients to Ask Questions: How to Overcome 'White-Coat Silence'," *Journal of the American Medical Association* 309, no. 22 (2013): 2325–2326.

44. See Chapter 4; "What You Need to Know," National Association of Professional Geriatric Care Managers, accessed October 21, 2014, http://www .caremanager.org/why-care-management/what-you-should-know/.

45. "John Hancock National Study Finds Long-Term Care Costs Continue to Climb across All Provider Options," *John Hancock News*, July 30, 2013, accessed November 1, 2014, http://www.johnhancock.com/about/news _details.php?fn=jul3013-text&yr=2013.

46. Paula Span, "Help by the Hour, or Less," *New York Times*, November 23, 2012, accessed November 1, 2014, http://newoldage.blogs.nytimes .com/2012/11/23/1123-help-by-the-hour/?_r=0.

CHAPTER 7

1. Richard W. Johnson and Janice S. Park, "Who Purchases Long-Term Care Insurance?" *Urban Institute Older Americans' Economic Security* 29 (March 2011), 1, accessed October 21, 2014, http://www.urban.org /UploadedPDF/412324-Long-Term-Care-Insurance.pdf; Jeffrey R. Brown and Amy Finkelstein, "Insuring Long-Term Care in the United States," *Journal of Economic Perspectives* 25, no. 4 (2011): 119.

2. *Statement of Thomas E. Hamilton, Director, Survey and Certification Group, Center for Medicaid and State Operations, Centers for Medicare & Medicaid Services on Making the Case for Long-Term Care Services and Supports Before the Senate Special Committee on Aging* (United States Senate, March 4, 2009), 7, accessed October 21, 2014, http://www .aging.senate.gov/imo/media/doc/hr205th.pdf.

3. Ibid., 8.

4. Beth Ann Swan, "A Nurse Learns Firsthand That You May Fend for Yourself After a Hospital Stay," *Health Affairs* 31, no. 11 (2012): 2579–2582.

5. Ibid.

6. Paula Span, *When the Time Comes: Families with Aging Parents Share Their Struggles and Solutions* (New York: Springboard Press, 2009), 161.

7. Anne Kelly et al., "Length of Stay for Older Adults Residing in Nursing Homes at the End of Life," *Journal of the American Geriatrics Society* 58, no. 9 (2010): 1703.

8. Brown and Finkelstein, "Insuring Long-Term Care in the United States," 122.

9. Span, *When the Time Comes*, 113.

10. "Average Number of Deficiencies per Certified Nursing Facility," Kaiser Family Foundation, accessed October 21, 2014, http://kff.org/other/state -indicator/avg-of-nursing-facility-deficiencies/.

11. "Percent of Certified Nursing Facilities with Top Ten Deficiencies," Kaiser Family Foundation, accessed October 21, 2014, http://kff.org/other/state-indicator/top-ten-nursing-facility-deficiencies/.

12. U.S. Department of Health and Human Services Office of Inspector General, *Adverse Events in Skilled Nursing Facilities: National Incidence among Medicare Beneficiaries* (Washington, DC: Office of Inspector General, 2014), 8, accessed October 21, 2014, http://oig.hhs.gov/oei/reports/oei-06-11-00370.pdf.

13. Span, *When the Time Comes*, 179–180.

14. Ibid., 184.

15. "Total Number of Residents in Certified Nursing Facilities, 2010," Kaiser Family Foundation, accessed October 21, 2014, http://www.statehealthfacts.org/comparemaptable.jsp?cat=8&ind=408 (providing state-by-state figures).

16. "Nursing Home Compare," Medicare.gov, accessed October 21, 2014, http://www.medicare.gov/nursinghomecompare/search.html.

17. See "Long-term Care Residential Options," Washington State Department of Social and Health Services, accessed October 21, 2014, http://www.altsa.dshs.wa.gov/pubinfo/housing/other/.

18. Editorial Board, "When Five-Star Care Is Substandard: Medicare's Flawed Ratings for Nursing Homes," *New York Times*, August 25, 2014, accessed November 2, 2014, http://www.nytimes.com/2014/08/26/opinion/medicares-flawed-ratings-for-nursing-homes.html?_r=0.

19. Span, *When the Time Comes*, 135.

20. Sudipto Banerjee, "Effects of Nursing Home Stays on Household Portfolios," *Employee Benefits Research Institute Issue Brief* 372 (2012), 9, accessed October 21, 2014, http://www.ebri.org/pdf/briefspdf/EBRI_IB_06-2012_No372_NrsHmStys.pdf.

21. "2012 Medicare Premiums, Deductibles and Co-Pays," Center for Medicare Advocacy, Inc., accessed October 21, 2014, http://www.medicareadvocacy.org/2012-medicare-premiums-deductibles-and-co-pays/; Centers for Medicare & Medicaid Services, *Medicare Coverage of Skilled Nursing Facility Care* (Baltimore, MD: Centers for Medicare & Medicaid Services, 2014), 18, accessed October 21, 2014, http://www.medicare.gov/Pubs/pdf/10153.pdf.

22. Paula Span, "Two Kinds of Hospital Patients: Admitted, and Not," *New York Times*, October 29, 2013, accessed October 21, 2014, http://newoldage.blogs.nytimes.com/2013/10/29/two-kinds-of-hospital-patients-admitted-and-not/.

23. Kelly April Tyrrell, "Delays, Controversy Muddle CMS' Two-Midnight Rule for Hospital Patient Admissions," *The Hospitalist*, April 2014, accessed November 2, 2014, http://www.the-hospitalist.org/details/article/6020631/Delays_Controversy_Muddle_CMS_Two-Midnight_Rule_for_Hospital_Patient_Admissions.html.

24. See Columbia Legal Services, "Questions and Answers on Medicaid for Nursing Home Residents," October 2012, accessed October 21, 2014, http://www.lawhelp.org/documents/1538915170EN.pdf?stateabbrev=/WA/.

25. Lawrence A. Frolik and Linda S. Whitton, *Everyday Law for Seniors* (Boulder, CO: Paradigm Publishers, 2012), 85–86.

26. 42 U.S.C. §1396p(c); "Medicaid's Asset Transfer Rules," ElderLaw-Answers, accessed November 2, 2014, http://www.elderlawanswers.com/medicaids-asset-transfer-rules-12015.

27. "Spousal Impoverishment," Medicaid.gov, accessed November 2, 2014, http://www.medicaid.gov/Medicaid-CHIP-Program-Information/By-Topics/Eligibility/Spousal-Impoverishment-Page.html;"MedicaidProtectionsforthe Healthy Spouse," ElderLawAnswers, accessed November 2, 2014, http://www.elderlawanswers.com/medicaid-protections-for-the-healthy-spouse-12019.

28. "Distribution of Certified Nursing Facility Residents by Primary Payer Source, 2010," Kaiser Family Foundation, accessed October 21, 2014, http://www.statehealthfacts.org/comparebar.jsp?ind=410&cat=8.

29. Banerjee, "Effects of Nursing Home Stays on Household Portfolios," 11.

30. Span, *When the Time Comes*, 115–116.

31. Christine Caffrey et al., "Residents Living in Residential Care Facilities: United States, 2010," *NCHS Data Brief* 91 (2012), 1, accessed October 21, 2014, http://www.cdc.gov/nchs/data/databriefs/db91.pdf.

32. Span, *When the Time Comes*, 117.

33. Ibid.

34. "John Hancock National Study Finds Long-Term Care Costs Continue to Climb across All Provider Options," *John Hancock News*, July 30, 2013, accessed November 25, 2014, http://www.johnhancock.com/about/news_details.php?fn=jul3013-text&yr=2013.

35. Span, *When the Time Comes*, 116.

36. Caffrey et al., "Residents Living in Residential Care Facilities: United States, 2010," 2.

37. Ibid.

38. Span, *When the Time Comes*, 130–131.

39. Ibid., 118; Sheryl Zimmerman et al., "How Good Is Assisted Living? Findings and Implications from an Outcomes Study," *Journal of Gerontology Series B Psychological Sciences & Social Science* 60, no. 4 (2005): S200–203.

40. See "Nursing Homes and Assisted Living," Office of the Minnesota Attorney General, accessed October 21, 2014, http://www.ag.state.mn.us/consumer/ylr/nursinghomesassistedliving.asp.

41. Nicholas Farber et al., *Aging in Place: A State Survey of Livability Policies and Practices*, National Conference of State Legislatures and the AARP Public Policy Institute, 2011, vii and 2, accessed October 21, 2014, http://www.ncsl.org/documents/transportation/Aging-in-Place-2011.pdf.

42. Span, *When the Time Comes*, 38.

43. See PA. STAT. ANN. Tit. 28 §§601.6 & 611.5.

44. *National Health Expenditures 2012 Highlights* (Baltimore, MD: Centers for Medicare & Medicaid Service), 1, accessed November 25, 2014, http://www.cms.gov/Research-Statistics-Data-and-Systems/Statistics-Trends-and-Reports/NationalHealthExpendData/downloads/highlights.pdf.

45. "Home Health Quality Initiative," Centers for Medicare & Medicaid Services, accessed November 25, 2014, https://www.cms.gov/Medicare/Quality-Initiatives-Patient-Assessment-Instruments/HomeHealthQualityInits/index.html?redirect=/HomeHealthQualityInits/.

46. "John Hancock National Study Finds Long-Term Care Costs Continue to Climb across All Provider Options."

47. Span, *When the Time Comes*, 43.

48. Tara Bahrampour, "D.C. Program Reflects National Trend toward Moving Older Americans Out of Nursing Homes," *Washington Post*, January 2, 2014, accessed October 21, 2014, http://www.washingtonpost.com/local/dc-program-reflects-national-trend-toward-moving-older-americans-out-of-nursing-homes/2014/01/02/8ac1a624-69c7-11e3-ae56-22de072140a2_story.html.

49. "Occupational Employment and Wages, May 2012, Home Health Aides," United States Department of Labor Bureau of Labor Statistics, accessed October 21, 2014, http://www.bls.gov/oes/current/oes311011.htm.

50. Paula Span, "A Better Way to Find Home Care Aides," *New York Times*, May 4, 2011 (quoting Dr. Dorie Seavey, director of policy research at P.H.I.), accessed October 21, 2014, http://newoldage.blogs.nytimes.com/2011/05/04/a-better-way-to-find-home-care-aides/.

51. Span, "A Better Way to Find Home Care Aides."

52. Span, *When the Time Comes*, 38–61.

53. Julianne Holt-Lunstad, Timothy B. Smith, and J. Bradley Layton, "Social Relationships and Mortality Risk: A Meta-Analytic Review," *PLoS Medicine* 7, no. 7 (2010): 14.

54. "Senior Centers: Fact Sheet," National Council on Aging, accessed October 21, 2014, http://www.ncoa.org/press-room/fact-sheets/senior-centers-fact-sheet.html.

55. "Statistics/Data," U.S. Department of Health and Human Services, National Center on Elder Abuse, Administration on Aging, accessed October 21, 2014, http://www.ncea.aoa.gov/Library/Data/index.aspx#problem.

56. "The National Voice for the Adult Day Service Community," National Adult Day Services Association, accessed October 21, 2014, http://www.nadsa.org/.

57. MetLife Mature Market Institute, National Adult Day Service Association, and Ohio State University College of Social Work, *The MetLife National Study of Adult Day Services: Providing Support to Individuals and Their*

Family Caregivers (New York: MetLife Mature Market Institute, 2010), 2–3, accessed October 21, 2014, https://www.metlife.com/assets/cao/mmi /publications/studies/2010/mmi-adult-day-services.pdf; Keith A. Anderson, Holly I. Dabelko-Schoeny, and Sarah D. Tarrant, "A Constellation of Concerns: Exploring the Present and the Future Challenges for Adult Day Services," *Home Health Care Management & Practice* 24, no. 3 (2012): 133.

58. "John Hancock National Study Finds Long-Term Care Costs Continue to Climb across All Provider Options."

59. Metlife Mature Market Institute et al., *The MetLife National Study of Adult Day Services*, 8.

60. "Site Visit Checklist," National Adult Day Services Association, accessed October 21, 2014, http://nadsa.org/consumers/site-visit-checklist/.

61. "State/International Association Partners," National Adult Day Services Association, accessed October 21, 2014, http://www.azularc.com /Development/nadsa/membership/state-association-partners/.

CHAPTER 8

1. June R. Lunney, Joanne Lynn, and Christopher Hogan, "Profiles of Older Medicare Decedents," *Journal of the American Geriatrics Society* 50, no. 6 (2002): 1108–1109. The other patients were classified as having died because of terminal illness (22 percent), organ system failure (16 percent), frailty (47 percent), or other causes.

2. June R. Lunney et al., "Patterns of Functional Decline at the End of Life," *Journal of the American Medical Association* 289, no. 18 (2003): 2388–2389. The others were categorized as dying of cancer (21 percent), organ failure (20 percent), frailty (20 percent), and other causes (24 percent).

3. *The Cambridge Edition of the Works of Jonathan Swift*, ed. Ian Gadd et al. (Cambridge: Cambridge University Press, 2012), 318–319.

4. Dena S. Davis, "Rational Suicide and Predictive Genetic Testing," *Journal of Clinical Ethics* 10, no. 4 (1999): 316–323.

5. "Facts and Figures," American Foundation for Suicide Prevention, accessed November 12, 2014, http://www.afsp.org/understanding-suicide /facts-and-figures.

6. Heike Baranzke, "'Sanctity-of-Life'—A Bioethical Principle for a Right to Life?," *Ethical Theory and Moral Practice* 15, no. 3 (2012): 296–302.

7. Or. Rev. Stat. Ann. Tit. 13, §§127.800–897; Wash. Rev. Code Ann. §§70.245.010–70.245.904; Vt. Stat. Ann. Tit. 18, §§5281–5292.

8. *Baxter v. State*, 224 P.3d 1211 (Mont. 2009).

9. "Oregon's Death with Dignity Act—2013," Oregon Public Health Division, accessed November 12, 2014, http://public.health.oregon.gov /ProviderPartnerResources/EvaluationResearch/DeathwithDignityAct /Documents/year16.pdf.

10. "Washington State Department of Health 2013 Death with Dignity Act Report," Washington State Department of Health, 1, accessed November 12, 2014, http://www.doh.wa.gov/portals/1/Documents/Pubs/422-109 -DeathWithDignityAct2013.pdf.

11. Katrina Hedberg and Susan Tolle, "Putting Oregon's Death with Dignity Act in Perspective: Characteristics of Decedents Who Did Not Participate," *Journal of Clinical Ethics* 20, no. 2 (2009): 133.

12. Ibid., 134.

13. "End-of-Life Consultation," Compassion & Choices, accessed October 21, 2014, https://www.compassionandchoices.org/what-we-do/end-of -life-counseling/.

14. Barbara Insley Crouch, "Toxicological Issues with Drugs Used to End Life," in *Drug Use in Assisted Suicide and Euthanasia*, ed. Margaret P. Battin and Arthur G. Lipman (Binghamton, NY: Haworth Press; 1996), 219.

15. "Accompanied Suicide," Dignitas, accessed October 21, 2014, http:// www.dignitas.ch/index.php?option=com_content&view=article&id=20&lan g=en.

16. Saskia Gauthier et al., "Suicide Tourism: A Pilot Study on the Swiss Phenomenon," *Journal of Medical Ethics* (first published online August 20, 2014): 1–7.

17. Zoe FitzGerald Carter, *Imperfect Endings: A Daughter's Story of Love, Loss, and Letting Go* (New York: Simon & Schuster, 2010); David Muller, "Physician-Assisted Death Is Illegal in Most States, so My Patient Made Another Choice," *Health Affairs* 31, no. 10 (2012): 2343–2346.

18. Paul T. Menzel and M. Colette Chandler-Cramer, "Advance Directives, Dementia, and Withholding Food and Water by Mouth," *Hastings Center Report* 44, no. 3 (2014): 33.

19. Rebecca Dresser, "Toward a Humane Death with Dementia," *Hastings Center Report* 44, no. 3 (2014): 39.

20. *Medicare Hospice Benefits* (Baltimore, MD: Centers for Medicare & Medicaid Services, 2013), 4, accessed October 21, 2014, http://www .medicare.gov/pubs/pdf/02154.pdf.

21. Kathleen A. Negri, "Advance Care Planning: The Attorney's Role in Helping Clients Achieve a 'Good Death'," *Colorado Lawyer* (July 2012): 71–72.

22. "The Model," National Center for Medical-Legal Partnership, accessed October 21, 2014, http://www.medical-legalpartnership.org/model.

23. "What Is Palliative Care?," American Academy of Hospice and Palliative Medicine, accessed October 21, 2014, http://www.aahpm.org/apps /blog/?p=1232.

24. Jennifer S. Temel et al., "Early Palliative Care for Patients with Metastatic Non–Small-Cell Lung Cancer," *New England Journal of Medicine* 363, no. 8 (2010): 738; Ravi B. Parikh et al., "Early Specialty Palliative Care—Translating

Data in Oncology into Practice," *New England Journal of Medicine* 369, no. 24 (2013): 2347.

25. *NHPCO's Facts and Figures: Hospice Care in America*, 2014 Edition (Alexandria, VA: National Hospice and Palliative Care Organization, 2014), 8, accessed November 5, 2014, http://www.nhpco.org/sites/default /files/public/Statistics_Research/2014_Facts_Figures.pdf.

26. Peter Whoriskey and Dan Keating, "Dying and Profits: The Evolution of Hospice," *The Washington Post*, December 26, 2014, accessed February 7, 2015, http://www.washingtonpost.com/business/economy/2014/12/26 /a7d90438-692f-11e4-b053-65cea7903f2e_story.html.

27. *Growth of Palliative Care in U.S. Hospitals 2013 Snapshot* (New York: Center to Advance Palliative Care, 2013), 1, accessed November 5, 2014, http://www.capc.org/capc-growth-analysis-snapshot-2013.pdf.

28. *Medicare Hospice Benefits*, 6–7.

29. Whoriskey and Keating, "Dying and Profits."

30. *Cruzan v. Director, Missouri Dept. of Health*, 497 U.S. 261 (1990).

31. Amy S. Kelley et al., "Determinants of Medical Expenditures in the Last 6 Months of Life," *Annals of Internal Medicine* 154, no. 4 (2011): 237.

32. Lisa R. Shugarman, Sandra L. Decker, and Anita Bercovitz, "Demographic and Social Characteristics and Spending at the End of Life," *Journal of Pain and Symptom Management* 38, no. 1 (2009): 16–17; Gerald F. Riley and James D. Lubitz, "Long-Term Trends in Medicare Payments in the Last Year of Life," *Health Services Research* 45, no. 2 (2010): 569 (finding an overall decrease "from 28.3 percent in 1978 to 25.1 percent in 2006").

33. Shugarman, Decker, and Bercovitz, "Demographic and Social Characteristics and Spending at the End of Life," 18–20.

34. Richard W. Johnson and Corina Mommaerts, *Will Health Care Costs Bankrupt Aging Boomers?* (Washington, DC: The Urban Institute, 2010); Allison K. Hoffman and Howell E. Jackson, "Retiree Out-of-Pocket Healthcare Spending: A Study of Consumer Expectations and Policy Implications," *American Journal of Law and Medicine* 39, no. 1 (2013): 73.

35. J. E. Wennberg et al., *Tracking the Course of Patients with Severe Chronic Illness: The Dartmouth Atlas of Health Care 2008* (Lebanon, NH: Dartmouth Institute for Health Policy & Clinical Practice, 2008), 83, accessed October 21, 2014, http://www.dartmouthatlas.org/downloads /atlases/2008_Chronic_Care_Atlas.pdf; Gerald W. Neuberg, "The Cost of End-of-Life Care: A New Efficiency Measure Falls Short of AHA /ACC Standards," *Cardiovascular Quality and Outcomes* 2, no. 2 (2009): 127.

36. Shannon Brownlee, *Overtreated: Why Too Much Medicine Is Making Us Sicker and Poorer* (New York: Bloomsbury, 2008), 205.

37. Ibid., 205–208.

38. Michael Wolff, "A Life Worth Ending," *New York Magazine*, May 20, 2012, accessed October 21, 2014, http://nymag.com/news/features /parent-health-care-2012-5/.

39. Michael S. Avidan and Alex S. Evers, "Review of Clinical Evidence for Persistent Cognitive Decline or Incident Dementia Attributable to Surgery or General Anesthesia," *Journal of Alzheimer's Disease* 24, no. 2 (2011): 202.

40. Wolff, "A Life Worth Ending."

41. Jonathan Rauch, "How Not to Die," *Atlantic*, April 24, 2013, accessed October 21, 2014, http://www.theatlantic.com/magazine/archive/2013/05 /how-not-to-die/309277/.

42. A. Coffey et al., "Nurses Preferred End-of-Life Treatment Choices in Five Countries," *International Nursing Review* 60, no. 3 (2013): 317–318.

43. Kelly Lauren Sloane, "If Only Grown-Ups Would Pay Attention," *Journal of American Medical Association* 309, no. 8 (2013): 780.

44. Rachel C. Carson et al., "Is Maximum Conservative Management an Equivalent Treatment Option to Dialysis for Elderly Patients with Significant Comorbid Disease?," *Clinical Journal of the American Society of Nephrology* 4, no. 10 (2009): 1618; Steven J. Baumrucker, "Ethics Roundtable," *American Journal of Hospice and Palliative Medicine* 22, no. 1 (2005): 61–65.

45. Wolff, "A Life Worth Ending."

46. See "Programs in Your State," Physician Orders for Life Sustaining Treatment Paradigm, accessed October 21, 2014, http://www.polst.org /programs-in-your-state/; Patricia A. Bomba, Marian Kemp, and Judith S. Black, "POLST: An Improvement Over Traditional Advance Directives," *Cleveland Clinic Journal of Medicine* 79, no. 7 (2012): 463.

47. Lawrence A. Frolik and Linda S. Whitton, Everyday Law for Seniors (Boulder, CO: Paradigm Publishers, 2012), 158.

48. Jeffrey P. Burns et al., "Do-Not-Resuscitate Order after 25 Years," *Critical Care Medicine* 31, no. 5 (2003): 1546; Jacqueline K. Yuen, M. Carrington Reid, and Michael D. Fetters, "Hospital Do-Not-Resuscitate Orders: Why They Have Failed and How to Fix Them," *Journal of General Internal Medicine* 26, no. 7 (2011): 792; Mary Catherine Beach and R. Sean Morrison, "The Effect of Do-Not-Resuscitate Orders on Physician Decision-Making," *Journal of the American Geriatrics Society* 50, no. 12 (2002): 2059; William J. Ehlenbach and J. Randall Curtis, "The Meaning of Do-Not-Resuscitation Orders: A Need for Clarity," *Critical Care Medicine* 39, no. 1 (2011): 193–194.

49. Rubin I. Cohen et al., "The Impact of Do-Not-Resuscitate Order on Triage Decisions to a Medical Intensive Care Unit," *Journal of Critical Care* 24, no. 2 (2009): 314.

50. Joline L. T. Chen et al., "Impact of Do-Not-Resuscitation Orders on Quality of Care Performance Measures in Patients Hospitalized with Acute Heart Failure," *Clinical Investigation* 156, no. 1 (2008): 80–82.

51. Derek K. Richardson et al., "The Impact of Early Do Not Resuscitate (DNR) Orders on Patient Care and Outcomes Following Resuscitation from Out of Hospital Cardiac Arrest," *Resuscitation* 84, no. 4 (2013): 486–487; Daniel J. Brauner, "What Should Lawyers Know about Advance Directives for Health Care? A Geriatrician Speaks Out," *Experience* 22, no. 3 (2013): 34–35.

52. Kathy L. Cerminara and Seth M. Bogin, "A Paper about a Piece of Paper: Regulatory Action as the Most Effective Way to Promote Use of Physician Orders for Life-sustaining Treatment," *Journal of Legal Medicine* 29, no. 4 (2008): 480.

53. Ibid., 484; Stanley A. Terman, "It Isn't Easy Being Pink: Potential Problems with POLST Paradigm Forms," *Hamline Law Review* 36, no. 2 (2013): 203.

54. Elliot N. Dorff, *Matters of Life and Death: A Jewish Approach to Modern Medical Ethics* (Philadelphia: Jewish Publication Society 1998), 199–200.

55. Robin Marantz Henig, "A Life or Death Situation," *New York Times Magazine*, July 17, 2013, 27.

56. Jaweed Kaleem, "Death Over Dinner, the Conversation Project Aim to Spark Discussions about the End of Life," *Huffington Post*, December 23, 2013, accessed October 21, 2014, http://www.huffingtonpost.com /2013/12/23/death-over-dinner-conversation-project_n_4495250.html.

57. "Views on End-of-Life Medical Treatments," *Pew Research Religion & Public Life Project*, November 21, 2013, accessed October 21, 2014, http:// www.pewforum.org/2013/11/21/views-on-end-of-life-medical-treatments/.

CHAPTER 9

1. Muriel R. Gillick, *The Denial of Aging: Perpetual Youth, Eternal Life, and Other Dangerous Fantasies* (Cambridge, MA: Harvard University Press, 2006), 257–258; Mayo Clinic Staff, "Mediterranean Diet: A Heart-Healthy Eating Plan," Mayo Clinic, accessed October 21, 2014, http:// www.mayoclinic.com/health/mediterranean-diet/CL00011; Fiona E. Matthews et al., on behalf of the Medical Research Council Cognitive Function and Ageing Collaboration, "A Two-Decade Comparison of Prevalence of Dementia in Individuals Aged 65 Years and Older from Three Geographical Areas of England: Results of the Cognitive Function and Ageing Study I and II," *Lancet* 382, no. 9902 (2013): 1410–1411, 6–7, accessed October 21, 2014, http://download.thelancet.com/flatcontentassets/pdfs /S0140673613615706.pdf; Ricardo Lopez, "Putting Off Retirement Cuts Chances of Dementia, Study Says," *Los Angeles Times*, July 15, 2013, accessed October 21, 2014, http://www.latimes.com/business/money/la-fi-mo -retirement-dementia-study-20130715,0,5992576.story.

2. Gillick, *The Denial of Aging*, 267.

3. See Chapter 2.

4. "Social Security Retirement Benefits," *Social Security Administration Publication* No. 05-10035 (April 2013), 4–14, accessed October 21, 2014, http://www.ssa.gov/pubs/EN-05-10035.pdf.

5. 42 U.S.C. §§3001–3057.

6. *Older Americans Act of 1965: Programs and Funding* (Washington, DC: National Health Policy Forum, 2012), 4–8, accessed October 21, 2014, http://www.nhpf.org/library/the-basics/Basics_OlderAmericansAct_02-23-12.pdf.

7. *S. 1562 Older Americans Act Reauthorization Act of 2013: As Reported by the Senate Committee on Health, Education, Labor, and Pensions on January 6* (Washington, DC: Congressional Budget Office Cost Estimate, 2014), 2, accessed October 21, 2014, http://www.cbo.gov/sites/default/files/s1562.pdf.

8. *Older Americans Act of 1965*, 5–6.

9. Susan M. Collins, Robbyn R. Wacker, and Karen A. Roberto, "Considering Quality of Life for Older Adults: A View from Two Countries," *Generations* 37, no. 1 (2013): 82–84; Adam Davey et al., "Life on the Edge: Patterns of Formal and Informal Help to Older Adults in the United States and Sweden," *Journals of Gerontology Series B Psychological Science and Social Science* 60, no. 5 (2005): S281–288.

10. See Chapter 5.

11. Ya-Huei Wu, Christine Fassert, and Anne-Sophie Rigaud, "Designing Robots for the Elderly: Appearance Issue and Beyond," *Archives of Gerontology and Geriatrics* 54, no. 1 (2012): 121.

12. Machiko R. Tomita et al., *Smart Home with Healthcare Technologies for Community-Dwelling Older Adults.* In Tech, 2010, 141–143, accessed October 21, 2014, http://cdn.intechopen.com/pdfs/9628/InTech-Smart_home_with_healthcare_technologies_for_community_dwelling_older_adults.pdf; Wolfram Ludwig et al., "Health-Enabling Technologies for the Elderly—An Overview of Services Based on a Literature Review," *Computer Methods and Programs in Biomedicine* 106, no. 2 (2012): 75–77; N. K. Suryadevara et al., "Sensor Data Fusion to Determine Wellness of an Elderly in Intelligent Home Monitoring Environment," *Instrumentation and Measurement Technology Conference (I2MTC), 2012 IEEE International* (2012): 947, accessed October 21, 2014; Julie Menack, "Technologies That Support Aging in Place," in *Handbook of Geriatric Care Management*, ed. Cathy Jo Cress (Burlington, MA: Jones & Bartlett Learning, 2011), 236.

13. Gillick, *The Denial of Aging*, 259.

14. Seongsu Kim and Daniel C. Feldman, "Working in Retirement: The Antecedents of Bridge Employment and Its Consequences for Quality of Life in Retirement," *Academy of Management Journal* 43, no. 6 (2000): 1206–1208.

15. Gillick, *The Denial of Aging*, 257; *Baby Boomers Retire* (Washington, DC: Pew Research Center, 2010), accessed October 21, 2014, http://www.pewresearch.org/daily-number/baby-boomers-retire.

16. Gillick, *The Denial of Aging*, 257.

17. *Angry Silents, Disengaged Millennials: The Generation Gap and the 2012 Election* (Washington, DC: Pew Research Center, 2011), 7, accessed October 21, 2014, http://www.people-press.org/files/legacy-pdf/11-3-11%20Generations%20Release.pdf.

18. Thom File, *The Diversifying Electorate—Voting Rates by Race and Hispanic Origin in 2012 (and Other Recent Elections)* (U.S. Census Bureau, 2013), 6, accessed October 21, 2014, http://www.census.gov/prod/2013pubs/p20-568.pdf; *America Goes to the Polls 2012: A Report of Voter Turnout in the 2012 Election* (Boston, MA: Nonprofit VOTE), 5, accessed October 21, 2014, http://www.nonprofitvote.org/voter-turnout.html.

19. Ibid.; Institute of Medicine, *Retooling for an Aging America: Building the Health Care Workforce* (Washington, DC: National Academies Press, 2008), 75–122.

20. "Medicare Primary Care Bonus Payment Program: Bonus Payment Program Overview," American College of Physicians, accessed October 21, 2014, http://www.acponline.org/running_practice/payment_coding/bonus.htm.

21. Melinda Abrams et al., *Realizing Health Reform's Potential: How the Affordable Care Act Will Strengthen Primary Care and Benefit Patients, Providers, and Payers* (Commonwealth Fund, 2011), 5–12, accessed October 21, 2014, http://www.commonwealthfund.org/~/media/Files/Publications/Issue%20Brief/2011/Jan/1466_Abrams_how_ACA_will_strengthen_primary_care_reform_brief_v3.pdf.

22. Gillick, *The Denial of Aging*, 257.

23. Menack, "Technologies That Support Aging in Place," 236–253; Younbo Jung et al., "Games for a Better Life: Effects of Playing Wii Games on the Well-Being of Seniors in a Long-Term Care Facility," *Proceedings of the Sixth Australasian Conference on Interactive Entertainment*, Article No. 5 (2009): 4–5.

24. Gillick, *The Denial of Aging*, 266.

Bibliography

20 C.F.R. §404.313 (2014).

20 C.F.R. §404.409 (2014).

42 CFR §§483.15-483.75 (2014).

42 U.S.C. §1395cc(f) (2011).

42 U.S.C. §1395i-3 (2014).

42 U.S.C. §1396p(c) (2010).

42 U.S.C §1396r (2011).

42 U.S.C §§3001-3057 (2014).

California Probate Code §4701, Part 3 (2014).

Consolidated Laws of New York §2983 (2012).

H.R. 3200, 11th Cong., 1st Sess. §1233 (2009).

Nursing Home Care Reform Act.

Older Americans Act of 1965.

Ohio Revised Code §1337.17 (2013).

Ohio Revised Code §2105.06 (2012), Statute of Descent and Distribution.

Ohio Revised Code 2135.07(B) (2013).

Or. Rev. Stat. Ann. Tit. 13, §§127.800-897 (2013).

Pa. Stat. Ann. Tit. 28 §§601.6 & 611.5 (2014).

Vt. Stat. Ann. Tit. 18, §§5281-5292 (2013).

Wash. Rev. Code Ann. §§70.245.010 – 70.245.904 (2009).

Baxter v. State, 224 P.3d 1211 (Mont. 2009).

Cruzan v. Director, Missouri Dept. of Health, 497 U.S. 261 (1990).

Health Care & Retirement Corp. of America v. Pittas, 46 A.3d 719 (Pa.Super. 2012).

AAA Association Communication. "Smart Features for Older Drivers." Accessed October 21, 2014. http://seniordriving.aaa.com/sites/default /files/Smart-Features-for-Older-Drivers-Brochure.pdf.

AAA Foundation for Traffic Safety. "Driver Medical Review Process / States WITH Medical Advisory Board (MAB)." Accessed October 21, 2014. http://lpp.seniordrivers.org/lpp/index.cfm?selection=statesMAB.

AAA Foundation for Traffic Safety. "Driver Medical Review Process / States WITHOUT Medical Advisory Board (MAB)." Accessed October 21, 2014. http://lpp.seniordrivers.org/lpp/index.cfm?selection=statesnoMAB.

AAA Foundation for Traffic Safety. "Family & Friend Reporting of At-Risk Drivers." Accessed October 21, 2014. http://lpp.seniordrivers.org/lpp /index.cfm?selection=reportingfamilyfriends1.

AAA Foundation for Traffic Safety. "How Family/Friends Report." Accessed October 21, 2014. http://lpp.seniordrivers.org/lpp/index.cfm?selection=re portingfamilyfriends2.

AAA Foundation for Traffic Safety. "Law Enforcement Reporting of At-Risk Drivers." Accessed October 21, 2014. http://lpp.seniordrivers.org/lpp /index.cfm?selection=lawenforcement.

AAA Foundation for Traffic Safety. "Physician Reporting of At-Risk Drivers." Accessed October 21, 2014. http://lpp.seniordrivers.org/lpp /index.cfm?selection=reportingdrs1&orderby=abbv&sortorder=asc&coun try=USA.

AAA Foundation for Traffic Safety. "Types of Conditions or Restrictions on Licenses." Accessed October 21, 2014. http://lpp.seniordrivers.org/lpp /index.cfm?selection=restrictedlicensetypes1.

AAA Senior Driving. Local Transportation Programs. Accessed October 20, 2014. http://dev.seniordriving.aaa.com/map.

AARP. "About Continuing Care Retirement Communities: What They Are and How They Work." Accessed October 20, 2014. http://www.aarp.org /relationships/caregiving-resource-center/info-09-2010/ho_continuing _care_retirement_communities.html.

AARP. "We Need to Talk: Family Conversation with Older Drivers, Module 2." Accessed October 21, 2014. http://www.aarp.org/home-garden /transportation/we_need_to_talk/?cmp=RDRCT-WNTT.

AARP. "What to Ask and Observe When Visiting Continuing Care Retirement Communities." Accessed October 20, 2014. http://www.aarp.org /relationships/caregiving-resource-center/info-09-2010/ho_what_to_ask _retirement_communities.html.

ABA Commission on Law and Aging. *Consumer's Tool Kit for Health Care Advance Planning,* 2nd ed. Washington, DC: American Bar Association on Law and Aging, 2005. Accessed October 20, 2014. http:// apps.americanbar.org/aging/publications/docs/consumer_tool_kit_bk .pdf.

Abrahms, Sally. "House Sharing for Boomer Women Who Would Rather Not Live Alone." *AARP Bulletin*, May 31, 2013. Accessed October 20, 2014. http://www.aarp.org/home-family/your-home/info-05-2013/older-women-roommates-house-sharing.html.

Abrams, Melinda, Rachel Nuzum, Stephanie Mika, and Georgette Lawlor. *Realizing Health Reform's Potential: How the Affordable Care Act Will Strengthen Primary Care and Benefit Patients, Providers, and Payers*. Commonwealth Fund, 2011. Accessed October 21, 2014. http://www.commonwealthfund.org/~/media/Files/Publications/Issue%20Brief/2011/Jan/1466_Abrams_how_ACA_will_strengthen_primary_care_reform_brief_v3.pdf.

Abrams, Robert. "Are You a Planner or a Gambler?" *New York State Bar Association Journal* 83, no. 6 (July–August 2011).

Alzheimer's Association. "2012 Alzheimer's Disease Facts and Figures." Accessed October 20, 2014. http://www.alz.org/downloads/facts_figures_2012.pdf.

Alzheimer's Association. "2014 Alzheimer's Disease Facts and Figures." Accessed November 10, 2014. http://www.alz.org/downloads/Facts_Figures_2014.pdf.

Amaria, Kainaz. "Long-Term Care Insurance: Who Needs It?" *NPR Special Series Family Matters: The Money Squeeze*, May 8, 2012. Accessed October 16, 2014. http://www.npr.org/2012/05/08/151970188/long-term-care-insurance-who-needs-it.

American Academy of Hospice and Palliative Medicine. "What Is Palliative Care?" Accessed October 21, 2014. http://www.aahpm.org/apps/blog/?p=1232.

American Association of Daily Money Managers. "ADMM's Certification Process—Frequently Asked Questions." Accessed October 16, 2014. http://www.aadmm.com/certification_faq.htm.

American Association of Daily Money Managers. "Code of Ethics." Accessed October 16, 2014. http://www.aadmm.com/code_of_ethics.htm.

American Association of Daily Money Managers. "DMMs and You." Accessed October 16, 2014. http://www.aadmm.com/dmms_and_you.htm.

American Association of Daily Money Managers. "Eligibility and Application Process for Professional Daily Money Manager Certification." Accessed October 16, 2014. http://www.aadmm.com/certification/14/pdmm_candidate_requirements_2014.pdf.

American Association of Daily Money Managers. "List of Certified Professional Daily Money Managers." Accessed November 25, 2014. http://www.aadmm.com/certification_list.htm.

American Association of Daily Money Managers. "Search for AADMM Members." Accessed November 9, 2014. http://www.aadmm.com/findDMM.php.

American Bar Association Commission on Law and Aging. "Consumer's Tool Kit for Health Care Advance Planning." Accessed December 1, 2014. http:// www.americanbar.org/groups/law_aging/resources/health_care_decision _making/consumer_s_toolkit_for_health_care_advance_planning.html.

American Bar Association Commission on Law and Aging. "Default Surrogate Consent Statutes" (June 2014). Accessed March 19, 2015. http:// www.americanbar.org/content/dam/aba/administrative/law_aging/2014 _default_surrogate_consent_statutes.authcheckdam.pdf.

American College of Physicians. "Medicare Primary Care Bonus Payment Program: Bonus Payment Program Overview." Accessed October 21, 2014. http://www.acponline.org/running_practice/payment_coding/bonus.htm.

American Foundation for Suicide Prevention. "Facts and Figures." Accessed November 12, 2014. http://www.afsp.org/understanding-suicide/facts-and -figures.

American Geriatrics Society. "FAQ's." Accessed October 20, 2014. http://www .americangeriatrics.org/advocacy_public_policy/gwps/gwps_faqs/id:3183.

American Hospital Association. "Advance Directive Notification." Accessed October 20, 2014. http://www.aha.org/content/13/piiw-walletcard.pdf.

American Hospital Association. "Put It in Writing: Questions and Answers on Advance Directives." 2012. Accessed October 20, 2014. http://www.aha .org/content/13/putitinwriting.pdf.

American Medical Association and National Highway Traffic and Safety Administration. *Physician's Guide to Assessing and Counseling Older Drivers*, 2nd ed. Chicago, IL: American Medical Association, 2010. Accessed November 4, 2014. http://www.aarp.org/content/dam/aarp /livable-communities/plan/transportation/older-drivers-guide.pdf.

Anderson, Diana. "Review of Advance Health Care Directive Laws in the United States, the Portability of Documents, and the Surrogate Decision Maker When No Document Is Executed." *National Academy of Elder Law Attorneys Journal* 8, no. 2 (2012): 183–203.

Anderson, Keith A., Holly I. Dabelko-Schoeny, and Sarah D. Tarrant. "A Constellation of Concerns: Exploring the Present and the Future Challenges for Adult Day Services." *Home Health Care Management & Practice* 24, no. 3 (2012): 132–139.

A Place for Mom. Accessed October 20, 2014. http://www.aplaceformom.com.

Area Agency on Aging. "What Is an Elder Law Attorney?" Accessed October 16, 2014. http://www.agingcarefl.org/aging/legal.

Assisted Living Federation of America. "Assisted Living Regulations and Licensing." Accessed October 20, 2014. http://www.alfa.org/alfa/State _Regulations_and_Licensing_Informat.asp.

Aulisio, Mark P., and Robert M. Arnold. "Role of the Ethics Committee: Helping to Address Value Conflicts or Uncertainties." *Chest* 134, no. 2 (2008): 417–424.

Avidan, Michael S., and Alex S. Evers. "Review of Clinical Evidence for Persistent Cognitive Decline or Incident Dementia Attributable to Surgery or General Anesthesia." *Journal of Alzheimer's Disease* 24, no. 2 (2011): 201–216.

Bahrampour, Tara. "D.C. Program Reflects National Trend toward Moving Older Americans Out of Nursing Homes." *Washington Post*, January 2, 2014. Accessed October 21, 2014. http://www.washingtonpost.com/local /dc-program-reflects-national-trend-toward-moving-older-americans-out -of-nursing-homes/2014/01/02/8ac1a624-69c7-11e3-ae56-22de072140a2 _story.html.

Ball, Karlene K., Daniel L. Roenker, Virginia G. Wadley, Jerri D. Edwards, David L. Roth, Gerald McGwin Jr., Robert Raleigh, John J. Joyce, Gayla M. Cissell, and Tina Dube. "Can High-Risk Older Drivers Be Identified Through Performance-Based Measures in a Department of Motor Vehicles Setting?" *Journal of the American Geriatrics Society* 54, no. 1 (2006): 77–84.

Banerjee, Sudipto. "Effects of Nursing Home Stays on Household Portfolios." *Employee Benefits Research Institute Issue Brief* 372 (2012). Accessed October 21, 2014. http://www.ebri.org/pdf/briefspdf/EBRI_IB_06-2012 _No372_NrsHmStys.pdf.

Bankrate. "Simple Savings Calculator." Accessed October 16, 2014. http:// www.bankrate.com/calculators/savings/simple-savings-calculator.aspx.

Baranzke, Heike. "'Sanctity-of-Life'—A Bioethical Principle for a Right to Life?" *Ethical Theory and Moral Practice* 15, no. 3 (2012): 295–308.

Baumrucker, Steven J. "Ethics Roundtable." *American Journal of Hospice and Palliative Medicine* 22, no. 1 (2005): 61–65.

Beach, Mary Catherine, and R. Sean Morrison. "The Effect of Do-Not-Resuscitate Orders on Physician Decision-Making." *Journal of the American Geriatrics Society* 50, no. 12 (2002): 2057–2061.

Behavioral Connections. "Advanced Directive Declaration for Mental Health Treatment." Accessed October 20, 2014. http://www.behavioralconnections .org/poc/view_doc.php?type=doc&id=8992.

Beiker, Sven A. "Legal Aspects of Autonomous Driving." *Santa Clara Law Review* 52, no. 4 (2012): 1145–1156.

Bekhet, Abir K., Jaclene A. Zauszniewski, and Wagdy E. Nakhla. "Reasons for Relocation to Retirement Communities: A Qualitative Study." *Western Journal of Nursing Research* 31, no. 4 (2009): 462–479.

Bernard, Tara Siegel. "Start-Up Aims to Bring Financial Planning to the Masses." *New York Times*, July 27, 2013. B1 & B4.

Block, Sandra. "Power of Attorney Can Be Valuable and Dangerous Tool." *USA Today*, December 8, 2008. Accessed October 20, 2014. http:// usatoday30.usatoday.com/money/perfi/columnist/block/2008 -12-08-managing-money-power-attorney_N.htm?csp=N009.

Board of Governors of the Federal Reserve. *Insights into the Financial Experiences of Older Adults: A Forum Briefing Paper.* Washington, DC: Board of Governors of the Federal Reserve System, 2013. Accessed November 12, 2014. http://www.federalreserve.gov/newsevents/conferences/older-adults-forum-paper-20130717.pdf.

Bomba, Patricia A., Marian Kemp, and Judith S. Black. "POLST: An Improvement Over Traditional Advance Directives." *Cleveland Clinic Journal of Medicine* 79, no. 7 (2012): 457–464.

Bragg, Elizabeth J., Gregg A. Warshaw, Karthikeyan Meganathan, and David E. Brewer. "The Development of Academic Geriatric Medicine in the United States 2005 to 2010: An Essential Resource for Improving the Medical Care of Older Adults." *Journal of the American Geriatrics Society* 60, no. 8 (2012): 1540–1545.

Brandon, Emily. "The Best Age to Buy Long-Term-Care Insurance." *U.S. News,* September 2, 2008. Accessed October 16, 2014. http://money.usnews.com/money/blogs/planning-to-retire/2008/09/02/the-best-age-to-buy-long-term-care-insurance.

Brauner, Daniel J. "What Should Lawyers Know About Advance Directives for Health Care? A Geriatrician Speaks Out." *Experience* 22, no. 3 (2013): 31–38.

Braver, E., and R. Trempel. "Are Older Drivers Actually at Higher Risk of Involvement in Collisions Resulting in Deaths or Non-fatal Injuries among Their Passengers and Other Road Users?" *Injury Prevention* 10, no. 1 (2004): 27–32.

Brodoff, Lisa. "Planning for Alzheimer's Disease with Mental Health Advance Directives." *Elder Law Journal* 17, no. 2 (2010): 239–308.

Brown, Alyssa. "Chronic Pain Rates Shoot Up Until Americans Reach Late 50s." *Gallup Wellbeing,* April 27, 2012. Accessed October 20, 2014. http://www.gallup.com/poll/154169/chronic-pain-rates-shoot-until-americans-reach-late-50s.aspx.

Brown, Jeffrey R., and Amy Finkelstein. "Insuring Long-Term Care in the United States." *Journal of Economic Perspective* 25, no. 4 (2011): 119–142.

Brown, Jeffrey R., Gopi Shah Goda, and Kathleen McGarry. "Long-Term Care Insurance Demand Limited by Beliefs about Needs, Concerns about Insurers, and Care Available from Family." *Health Affairs* 31, no. 6 (2012): 1294–1302.

Brownlee, Shannon. *Overtreated: Why too Much Medicine Is Making Us Sicker and Poorer.* New York: Bloomsbury, 2007.

Burns, Jeffrey P., Jeffrey Edwards, Judith Johnson, Ned H. Cassem, and Robert D. Truog. "Do-Not-Resuscitate Order after 25 Years." *Critical Care Medicine* 31, no. 5 (2003): 1543–1550.

Caffrey, Christine, Manisha Sengupta, Eunice Park-Lee, Abigail Moss, Emily Rosenoff, and Lauren Harris-Kojetin. "Residents Living in Residential

Care Facilities: United States, 2010." *NCHS Data Brief* 91 (2012). Accessed October 21, 2014. http://www.cdc.gov/nchs/data/databriefs/db91.pdf.

California Advocates for Nursing Home Reform. *Points to Consider for CCRC Consumers*. San Francisco, CA: CANHR, 2009. Accessed October 20, 2014. http://canhr.org/publications/PDFs/CCRCPtsToConsider.pdf.

California's Three-Tier Driving-Centered Assessment System: Outcome Analysis. State of California Department of Motor Vehicles, 2011. Accessed October 21, 2014. http://apps.dmv.ca.gov/about/profile/rd/r_d_report/Section_2/S2 -234.pdf.

Campbell, John Y., Samuel C. Durso, Lynsey E. Brandt, Thomas E. Finucane, and Peter M. Abadir. "The Unknown Profession: A Geriatrician." *Journal of the American Geriatrics Society* 61, no. 3 (2013): 447–449.

Cantheclutter. Accessed October 16, 2014. http://cantheclutter.com/.

CARF-CCAC. *Consumer Guide to Understanding Financial Performance and Reporting in Continuing Care Retirement Communities*. Washington, DC: CARF-CCAC, 2007. Accessed October 20, 2014. http://www.carf.org /FinancialPerformanceCCRCs/.

CARF International. "List of CARF-CCAC Accredited Continuing Care Retirement Communities (2014)." Accessed November 20, 2014. http:// carf.org/ccrcListing.aspx.

Caring.com Staff. "Geriatric Care Managers." Accessed October 16, 2014. http://www.caring.com/local/geriatric-care-managers.

Carrns, Ann. "Save for Retirement First, the Children's Education Second." *New York Times*, March 1, 2014. B4.

Carson, Rachel C., Maciej Juszczak, Andrew Davenport, and Aine Burns. "Is Maximum Conservative Management an Equivalent Treatment Option to Dialysis for Elderly Patients with Significant Comorbid Disease?" *Clinical Journal of the American Society of Nephrology* 4, no. 10 (2009): 1611–1619.

Carter, Zoe FitzGerald. *Imperfect Endings: A Daughter's Story of Love, Loss, and Letting Go*. New York: Simon & Schuster, 2010.

Center for Medicare Advocacy, Inc. "2012 Medicare Premiums, Deductibles and Co-Pays." Accessed October 21, 2014. http://www.medicareadvocacy .org/2012-medicare-premiums-deductibles-and-co-pays/.

Center for Workforce Studies Association of American Medical Colleges. *Recent Studies and Reports on Physician Shortages in the US* (AAMC, 2012). Accessed October 21, 2014. https://www.aamc.org/download/100598/data /recentworkforcestudies.pdf.

Centers for Disease Control and Prevention. "Older Adult Drivers: Get the Facts." Accessed October 21, 2014. http://www.cdc.gov/Motorvehiclesafety /Older_Adult_Drivers/adult-drivers_factsheet.html.

Centers for Disease Control and Prevention. "Therapeutic Drug Use." *Fast-Stats*. Accessed November 20, 2014. http://www.cdc.gov/nchs/fastats /drug-use-therapeutic.htm.

Centers for Medicare & Medicaid Services. "Home Health Quality Initiative." Accessed November 25, 2014. https://www.cms.gov/Medicare/Quality -Initiatives-Patient-Assessment-Instruments/HomeHealthQualityInits /index.html?redirect=/HomeHealthQualityInits/.

Centers for Medicare & Medicaid Services. *Medicare Coverage of Skilled Nursing Facility Care*. Baltimore, MD: Centers for Medicare & Medicaid Services, 2014. Accessed October 21, 2014. http://www.medicare.gov /Pubs/pdf/10153.pdf.

Centers for Medicare & Medicaid Services. *Medicare Hospice Benefits*. Baltimore, MD: Centers for Medicare & Medicaid Services, 2013. Accessed October 21, 2014. http://www.medicare.gov/pubs/pdf/02154.pdf.

Centers for Medicare & Medicaid Service. *National Health Expenditures 2012 Highlights*. Baltimore, MD: Centers for Medicare & Medicaid Service. Accessed November 25, 2014. http://www.cms.gov/Research-Statistics-Data -and-Systems/Statistics-Trends-and-Reports/NationalHealthExpendData /downloads/highlights.pdf.

Center to Advance Palliative Care. *Growth of Palliative Care in U.S. Hospitals 2013 Snapshot*. New York: Center to Advance Palliative Care, 2013. Accessed November 5, 2014. http://www.capc.org/capc-growth-analysis -snapshot-2013.pdf.

Cerminara, Kathy L., and Seth M. Bogin. "A Paper about a Piece of Paper: Regulatory Action as the Most Effective Way to Promote Use of Physician Orders for Life-sustaining Treatment." *Journal of Legal Medicine* 29, no. 4 (2008): 479–503.

Chen, Joline L. T., Jonathan Sosnov, Darleen Lessard, and Robert J. Goldberg. "Impact of Do-Not-Resuscitation Orders on Quality of Care Performance Measures in Patients Hospitalized with Acute Heart Failure." *Clinical Investigation* 156, no. 1 (2008): 78–84.

Cheung, Ivan, and Anne T. McCartt. "Declines in Fatal Crashes of Older Drivers: Changes in Crash Risk and Survivability." *Accident Analysis and Prevention* 43, no. 3 (2011): 666–674.

Choose to Save. "Ballpark E$timate." Accessed October 16, 2014. http://www .choosetosave.org/ballpark/index.cfm?fa=interactive.

Christensen, Kaare, Mikael Thinggaard, Anna Oksuzyan, Troels Steenstrup, Karen Andersen-Ranberg, Bernard Jeune, Matt McGue, and James W. Vaupel. "Physical and Cognitive Functioning of People Older Than 90 Years: A Comparison of Two Danish Cohorts Born 10 Years Apart." *Lancet* 382, no. 9903 (2013): 1507–1513.

Clark, Peter A., Jill R. Friedman, David W. Crosson, and Matthew Fadus. "Concierge Medicine: Medical, Legal and Ethical Perspectives." *Internet Journal of Law, Healthcare and Ethics* 7, no. 1 (2011): 1–38.

Cleveland Clinic. "State of Ohio Health Care Power of Attorney." Accessed October 20, 2014. http://my.clevelandclinic.org/Documents/Patients/health -care-power-of-attorney-form.pdf.

Cleveland Clinic. "State of Ohio Living Will Declaration." Accessed October 20, 2014. http://my.clevelandclinic.org/ccf/media/Files/Patients/OhioLivingWill.pdf.

Coffey, A., G. McCarthy, E. Weathers, M. I. Friedman, K. Gallo, M. Ehrenfeld, M. Itzhaki, S. Chan, W. H. Li, P. Poletti, R. Zanotti, D. W. Molloy, C. McGlade, and J. J. Fitzpatrick. "Nurses Preferred End-of-Life Treatment Choices in Five Countries." *International Nursing Review* 60, no. 3 (2013): 313–319.

Cohen, Rubin I., Gita N. Lisker, Ann Eichorn, Alan S. Multz, and Alan Silver. "The Impact of Do-Not-Resuscitate Order on Triage Decisions to a Medical Intensive Care Unit." *Journal of Critical Care* 24, no. 2 (2009): 311–315.

Colby, Sandra L., and Jennifer M. Ortman. "The Baby Boom Cohort in the United States: 2012 to 2060: Population Estimates and Projections." *United States Census Bureau Report* P25-1141, May 2014. Accessed November 7, 2014. http://www.census.gov/prod/2014pubs/p25-1141.pdf.

Collins, Susan M., Robbyn R. Wacker, and Karen A. Roberto. "Considering Quality of Life for Older Adults: A View from Two Countries." *Generations* 37, no. 1 (2013): 80–86.

Columbia Legal Services. *Questions and Answers on Medicaid for Nursing Home Residents.* October 2012. Accessed October 21, 2014. http://www.lawhelp.org/documents/1538915170EN.pdf?stateabbrev=/WA/.

Compassion & Choices. "End-of-Life Consultation." Accessed October 21, 2014. https://www.compassionandchoices.org/what-we-do/end-of-life-counseling/.

Cress, Cathy Jo. *Handbook of Geriatric Care Management*, 3rd ed. Burlington, MA: Jones & Bartlett Learning, 2012.

Crooks, Valerie C., James Lubben, Diana B. Petitti, Deborah Little, and Vicki Chiu. "Social Network, Cognitive Function, and Dementia Incidence among Elderly Women." *American Journal of Public Health* 98, no. 7 (2008): 1221–1227.

Cropp, Ian. "Why Do Hearing Aids Cost So Much?" *AARP Bulletin*, May 5, 2011. Accessed October 16, 2014. http://www.aarp.org/health/conditions-treatments/info-05-2011/hearing-aids-cost.html.

Crouch, Barbara Insley. "Toxicological Issues with Drugs Used to End Life." In *Drug Use in Assisted Suicide and Euthanasia*, edited by Margaret P. Battin and Arthur G. Lipman, 211–222. Binghamton, NY: Haworth Press, 1996.

Davey, Adam, Elia E. Femia, Steven H. Zarit, Dennis G. Shea, Gerdt Sundström, Stig Berg, Michael A. Smyer, and Jyoti Savla. "Life on the Edge: Patterns of Formal and Informal Help to Older Adults in the United States and Sweden." *Journals of Gerontology Series B Psychological Science & Social Science* 60, no. 5 (2005): S281–S288.

Davis, Dena S. "Rational Suicide and Predictive Genetic Testing." *Journal of Clinical Ethics* 10, no. 4 (1999): 316–323.

Define by Redesign. "The Basics of Home Staging." Accessed October 16, 2014. http://www.definebyredesign.com/services/homestaging.php.

DeGood, Kevin, David Goldberg, Nick Donohue, and Lilly Shoup. *Aging in Place, Stuck without Options: Fixing the Mobility Crisis Threatening the Baby Boom Generation*. Transportation for America, 2011. Accessed October 21, 2014. http://t4america.org/docs/SeniorsMobilityCrisis.pdf.

Desapriya, Ediriweera, Harshani Wijeratne, Sayed Subzwari, Shelina Babul-Wellar, Kate Turcotte, Fahra Rajabali, Jacqueline Kinney, and Ian Pike. "Vision Screening of Older Drivers for Preventing Road Traffic Injuries and Fatalities." *Cochrane Database of Systematic Reviews* 2 (2014): CD006252.

Didion, Joan. *Blue Nights*. New York: Vintage, 2011.

Dignitas. "Accompanied Suicide." Accessed October 21, 2014. http://www .dignitas.ch/index.php?option=com_content&view=article&id=20&lang=en.

Dorff, Elliot N. *Matters of Life and Death: A Jewish Approach to Modern Medical Ethics*. Philadelphia: Jewish Publication Society, 1998.

Dresser, Rebecca. "Dworkin on Dementia: Elegant Theory, Questionable Policy." *Hastings Center Report* 25, no. 6 (1995): 32–38.

Dresser, Rebecca. "Missing Persons: Legal Perceptions of Incompetent Patients." *Rutgers Law Review* 46, no. 2 (1994): 609–719.

Dresser, Rebecca. "Toward a Humane Death with Dementia." *Hastings Center Report* 44, no. 3 (2014): 38–40.

Duckworth, Ken. *Depression in Older Persons Fact Sheet*. National Alliance on Mental Illness, 2009. Accessed October 20, 2014. http://www.nami .org/Content/NavigationMenu/Mental_Illnesses/Depression/Depression _Older_Persons_FactSheet_2009.pdf.

Dworkin, Ronald. *Life's Dominion: An Argument about Abortion, Euthanasia, and Individual Freedom*. New York: Vintage, 1994.

Ebeling, Ashlea. "Continuing Care Communities: A Big Investment with Catches." *Forbes*, September 26, 2011. Accessed October 20, 2014. http://www.forbes.com/sites/ashleaebeling/2011/09/26/continuing-care -communities-a-big-investment-with-catches/.

Eberhard, John. "Older Drivers' 'High Per-Mile Crash Involvement': The Implications for Licensing Authorities." *Traffic Injury Prevention* 9, no. 4 (2008): 284–290.

Ehlenbach, William J., and J. Randall Curtis. "The Meaning of Do-Not-Resuscitation Orders: A Need for Clarity." *Critical Care Medicine* 39, no. 1 (2011): 193–194.

ElderLawAnswers. "Medicaid's Asset Transfer Rules." Accessed November 2, 2014. http://www.elderlawanswers.com/medicaids-asset-transfer-rules-12015.

ElderLawAnswers. "Medicaid Protections for the Healthy Spouse." Accessed November 2, 2014. http://www.elderlawanswers.com/medicaid -protections-for-the-healthy-spouse-12019.

Emling, Shelley. "Study Shows Surprising Number of Drivers Over 100." *The Huffington Post*, September 23, 2013. Accessed October 21, 2014. http://www.huffingtonpost.com/2013/09/23/older-drivers_n_3975579.html.

Enguidanos, Susan M., and Paula M. Jamison. "Moving from Tacit Knowledge to Evidence-Based Practice: The Kaiser Permanente Community Partners Study." *Home Health Care Service Quarterly* 25, no. 1–2 (2006): 13–31.

Erickson, Mary Ann, Donna Dempster-McClain, Carol Whitlow, and Phyllis Moen. "Social Integration and the Move to a Continuing Care Retirement Community." In *Social Integration in the Second Half of Life*, edited by Karl Pillemer, Phyllis Moen, Elaine Wethington, and Nina Glasgow, 211–227. Baltimore, MD: Johns Hopkins University Press, 2000.

Ertel, Karen, Maria Glymour, and Lisa F. Berkman. "Effects of Social Integration on Preserving Memory Function in a Nationally Representative US Elderly Population." *American Journal of Public Health* 98, no. 7 (2008): 1215–1220.

Farber, Nicholas, Douglas Shinkle, with Jana Lynott, Wendy Fox-Grage, and Rodney Harrell. *Aging in Place: A State Survey of Livability Policies and Practices*. National Conference of State Legislatures and the AARP Public Policy Institute, 2011. Accessed October 21, 2014. http://www.ncsl.org/documents/transportation/Aging-in-Place-2011.pdf.

Federal Highway Administration. "Distribution of Licensed Drivers—2012: By Sex and Percentage in Each Age Group and Relation to Population Table DL-20." In Office of Highway Policy Information. *Highway Statistics 2012*. Washington, DC: Federal Highway Administration, 2014. DL-20. Accessed November 25, 2014. http://www.fhwa.dot.gov/policyinformation/statistics/2012/index.cfm.

Federal Interagency Forum on Aging Related Statistics. "Population." Accessed October 16, 2014. http://www.agingstats.gov/Main_Site/Data/2012_Documents/Population.aspx.

Federal Trade Commission. "Funeral Costs and Pricing Checklist." Accessed October 20, 2014. http://www.consumer.ftc.gov/articles/0301-funeral-costs-and-pricing-checklist#Calculating.

Fifth Third Bank. "Is Opening a Roth IRA Right for You?" Accessed October 16, 2014. https://www.53.com/site/personal-banking/investments/our-solutions/rsp-roth-iras.html.

File, Thom. *The Diversifying Electorate—Voting Rates by Race and Hispanic Origin in 2012 (and Other Recent Elections)*. United States Census Bureau, 2013. Accessed October 21, 2014. http://www.census.gov/prod/2013pubs/p20-568.pdf.

Financial Planning Association. "Pro Bono." Accessed October 16, 2014. http://www.onefpa.org/advocacy/Pages/ProBonoProgram.aspx.

Financial Planning Association Connecticut. "FPA CT Pro Bono Network." Accessed October 16, 2014. http://fpact.org/net/home/ProBono/FpaCtProBonoNetwork.pdf.

Fiori, Katherine L., Toni C. Antonucci, and Kai S. Cortina. "Social Network Typologies and Mental Health among Older Adults." *Journal of Gerontology: Series B* 61, no. 1 (2006): 25–32.

Fiscella, Kevin, and Ronald M. Epstein. "So Much to Do, So Little Time: Care for the Socially Disadvantaged and the 15-Minute Visit." *Archives of Internal Medicine* 168, no. 17 (2008): 1843–1852.

Freid, Virginia M., Amy B. Bernstein, and Mary Ann Bush. "Multiple Chronic Conditions among Adults Aged 45 and Over: Trends Over the Past 10 Years." *NCHS Data Brief* 100 (July 2012). Accessed October 16, 2014. http://www.cdc.gov/nchs/data/databriefs/db100.pdf.

French, Michael T., Jenny F. Homer, Shay Klevay, Edward Goldman, Steven G. Ullmann, and Barbara E. Kahn. "Is the United States Ready to Embrace Concierge Medicine?" *Population Health Management* 13, no. 4 (2010): 177–182.

Frolik, Lawrence A., and Linda S. Whitton. *Everyday Law for Seniors: Updated with the Latest Federal Benefits.* Boulder, CO: Paradigm Publishers, 2012.

Frongillo, Edward A., Tanushree D. Isaacman, Claire M. Horan, Elaine Wethington, and Karl Pillemer. "Adequacy of and Satisfaction with Delivery and Use of Home-Delivered Meals." *Journal of Nutrition for the Elderly* 29, no. 3 (2010): 211–226.

Frongillo, Edward A., and Wendy S. Wolfe. "Impact of Participation in Home-Delivered Meals on Nutrient Intake, Dietary Patterns, and Food Insecurity of Older Persons in New York State." *Journal of Nutrition for the Elderly* 29, no. 3 (2010): 293–310.

Fry, Sara T., Dennis C. Cunningham, Jacqueline Fajkowski, Mary McCormick-Gendzel, and Christine Day. "Evolution of a Home Health Ethics Committee." *Home Healthcare Nurse* 19, no. 9 (2001): 565–570.

Gadd, Ian, Ian Higgins, James McLaverty, Claude Rawson, Valerie Rumbold, and Abigail Williams, eds. *The Cambridge Edition of the Works of Jonathan Swift.* Cambridge: Cambridge University Press, 2012.

Gauthier, Saskia, Julian Mausbach, Thomas Reisch, and Christine Bartsch. "Suicide Tourism: A Pilot Study on the Swiss Phenomenon." *Journal of Medical Ethics* (first published online August 20, 2014): 1–7. Accessed January 24, 2015. http://www.west-info.eu/the-europeans-who-choose-suicide-tourism/medethics-2014-102091-full/.

Gawande, Atul. "The Way We Age Now." *New Yorker,* April 30, 2007. Accessed October 20, 2014. http://www.newyorker.com/magazine/2007/04/30/the-way-we-age-now.

Gillick, Muriel R. *The Denial of Aging: Perpetual Youth, Eternal Life, and Other Dangerous Fantasies*. Cambridge, MA: Harvard University Press, 2006.

Gillispie, Mark. "Driver in Fatal Hit-Skip Avoids Prison Time." *Cleveland Plain Dealer*, January 15, 2013, B3.

Glasgow, Nina. "An Intervention to Improve Transportation Arrangements." In *Social Integration in the Second Half of Life*, edited by Karl Pillemer, Phyllis Moen, Elaine Wethington, and Nina Glasgow, 247–264. Baltimore, MD: Johns Hopkins University Press, 2000.

Gleckman, Howard. "Should You Buy Long-Term Care Insurance? Maybe Not." *Forbes*, January 18, 2012. Accessed October 16, 2014. http://www.forbes.com/sites/howardgleckman/2012/01/18/should-you-buy-long-term-care-insurance-maybe-not/.

Golden Girls Network. Accessed October 20, 2014. http://goldengirlsnetwork.com/.

Goreman, Chandra C., Lisa E. Tucker, Jennifer Flynn, and Michael West. *Senior Transportation Alternatives: Why Are They Important and What Makes Them Work?* Tampa, FL: NCTR at CUTR, 2003. Accessed October 21, 2014. http://www.nctr.usf.edu/pdf/473-09.pdf.

Gottschalk, Andrew, and Susan A. Flocke. "Time Spent in Face-to-Face Patient Care and Work Outside the Examination Room." *Annals of Family Medicine* 3, no. 6 (2005): 488–493.

Grabowski, David C., Christine M. Campbell, and Michael A. Morrisey. "Elderly Licensure Laws and Motor Vehicle Fatalities." *Journal of the American Medical Association* 291, no. 23 (2004): 2840–2846.

Graham, Judith. "A Choice of Community Care, in Your Own Home." *New York Times*, September 17, 2012. Accessed October 20, 2014. http://newoldage.blogs.nytimes.com/2012/09/17/a-choice-of-community-care-but-in-your-own-home/.

Greene, Kelly. "Long-Term Care: What Now?" *Wall Street Journal*, March 9, 2012. Accessed October 16, 2014. http://online.wsj.com/articles/SB10001424052970203961204577269842991276650.

Groger, Lisa, and Jennifer Kinney. "CCRC Here We Come! Reasons for Moving to a Continuing Care Retirement Community." *Journal of Housing for the Elderly* 20, no. 4 (2006): 79–101.

Gross, Jane. "Doctor Focuses on the Minds of the Elderly." *New York Times*, April 30, 2011. Accessed October 20, 2014. http://www.nytimes.com/2011/05/01/us/01elderly.html?pagewanted=all.

Gruenewald, Tara L., Arun S. Karlamangla, Gail A. Greendale, Burton H. Singer, and Teresa E. Seeman. "Increased Mortality Risk in Older Adults with Persistently Low or Declining Feelings of Usefulness to Others." *Journal of Aging Health* 21, no. 2 (2009): 398–425.

Hamilton, Martha M. "What Health Care Will Cost You." *AARP Bulletin*, January–February 2013. Accessed October 31, 2014. http://www
.aarp.org/health/medicare-insurance/info-12-2012/health-care-costs
.html.

Harris-Kojetin, Lauren, Manisha Sengupta, Eunice Park-Lee, and Roberto Valverde. *Long-Term Care Services in the United States: 2013 Overview.* Hyattsville, MD: National Center for Health Statistics, 2013. Accessed November 7, 2014. http://www.cdc.gov/nchs/data/nsltcp/long_term_care
_services_2013.pdf.

Healthinaging.org. "Geriatrics Basic Facts & Information." Accessed October 20, 2014. http://www.healthinaging.org/aging-and-health-a-to-z
/topic:geriatrics/.

Hedberg, Katrina, and Susan Tolle. "Putting Oregon's Death with Dignity Act in Perspective: Characteristics of Decedents Who Did Not Participate." *Journal of Clinical Ethics* 20, no. 2 (2009): 133–135.

Helman, Ruth, Nevin Adams, Craig Copeland, and Jack VanDerhei. "The 2014 Retirement Confidence Survey: Confidence Rebounds—for Those With Retirement Plans." *Employee Benefit Research Institute Brief* 397 (2014). Accessed October 23, 2014. http://www.ebri.org/pdf/briefspdf
/EBRI_IB_397_Mar14.RCS.pdf.

Helman, Ruth, Craig Copeland, and Jack VanDerhei. "The 2012 Retirement Confidence Survey: Job Insecurity, Debt Weigh on Retirement, Confidence, Savings." *Employee Benefit Research Institute Brief* 369 (2012). Accessed October 16, 2014. http://www.ebri.org/pdf/surveys/rcs/2012
/EBRI_IB_03-2012_No369_RCS.pdf.

Henig, Robin Marantz. "A Life or Death Situation." *New York Times Magazine*, July 17, 2013, 27.

Hessels, Virginia, Glenn S. Le Prell, and William C. Mann. "Advances in Personal Emergency Response and Detection Systems." *Assistive Technology* 23, no. 3 (2011): 152–166.

Highway Loss Data Institute. "Estimating the Effect of Projected Changes in the Driving Population on Collision Claim Frequency." *Highway Loss Data Institute Bulletin* 29, no. 8 (2012). Accessed October 21, 2014. http://
www.iihs.org/research/topics/pdf/HLDI_bulletin_29.8.pdf.

Hoffman, Allison K., and Howell E. Jackson. "Retiree Out-of-Pocket Healthcare Spending: A Study of Consumer Expectations and Policy Implications." *American Journal of Law and Medicine* 39, no. 1 (2013): 1–72.

Hoffman, Sharona, and Andy Podgurski. "E-Health Hazards: Provider Liability and Electronic Health Record Systems." *Berkeley Technology Law Journal* 24, no. 4 (2010): 1524–1581.

Holt-Lunstad, Julianne, Timothy B. Smith, and J. Bradley Layton. "Social Relationships and Mortality Risk: A Meta-Analytic Review." *PLoS Medicine* 7, no. 7 (2010): 1–20.

Institute for Oral Health 2008 Focus Group #1 on "Oral Health in Aging America." *Oral Health Needs for Seniors: Challenges and Solutions in Dental Care for Aging Adults.* Institute for Oral Health, 2008. Accessed October 21, 2014. http://iohwa.org/2008fg/IOHFeb08FocusGroup_whitepaper.pdf.

Institute of Medicine. *Retooling for an Aging America: Building the Health Care Workforce.* Washington, DC: National Academies Press, 2008.

Institute of Medicine. "Statement of John W. Rowe Before the Special Committee on Aging, U.S. Senate" (April 16, 2008). Accessed October 21, 2014. http://www.iom.edu/~/media/Files/Report%20Files/2008/Retooling-for-an-Aging-America-Building-the-Health-Care-Workforce/Statement%20of%20John%20W%20Rowe%20MD%20Before%20the%20Special%20Committee%20on%20Aging%20US%20Senate%20April%2016%202008.pdf.

Insurance Institute for Highway Safety. "Older Drivers: November 2014." Accessed November 12, 2014. http://www.iihs.org/iihs/topics/laws/olderdrivers.

Insurance Institute for Highway Safety. "Q&A: Older Drivers." Last modified March 2014. Accessed November 26, 2014. http://www.iihs.org/iihs/topics/t/older-drivers/qanda.

Intelius. Accessed October 20, 2014. https://www.intelius.com/.

International Association of Home Staging Professionals. Accessed October 20, 2014. http://www.iahsp.com.

Jacobs, Deborah L. "How to Do Estate Planning on the Cheap." *Forbes,* November 19, 2010. Accessed October 20, 2014. http://www.forbes.com/forbes/2010/1206/investment-guide-living-will-software-cheap-estate-planning.html.

J.D. Power. "2014 Mercedes-Benz E-Class Introduces 'Intelligent Drive'." December 17, 2012. Accessed October 21, 2014. http://autos.jdpower.com/content/blog-post/apv6Qyy/2014-mercedes-benz-e-class-introduces-intelligent-drive.htm.

Jenkins, Kristi Rahrig, Amy Mehraban Pienta, and Ann L. Horgas. "Activity and Health-Related Quality of Life in Continuing Care Retirement Communities." *Research on Aging* 24 (2002): 124–149.

Jenness, James W., Neil D. Lerner, Steve Mazor, J. Scott Osberg, and Brian C. Tefft. *Use of Advanced In-Vehicle Technology by Young and Older Early Adopters: Survey Results on Adaptive Cruise Control Systems* (March 2008), Report No. DOT HS 810 917. Washington, DC: National Highway Traffic Safety Administration, 2008.

Jeste, Dilip V. "Aging and Mental Health: Bad News and Good News." *Psychiatric News* (from the American Psychiatric Association), July 6, 2012. Accessed November 6, 2014. http://psychnews.psychiatryonline.org/doi/full/10.1176/pn.47.13.psychnews_47_13_3-a.

John Hancock News. "John Hancock National Study Finds Long-Term Care Costs Continue to Climb across All Provider Options." July 30, 2013. Accessed November 1, 2014. http://www.johnhancock.com/about/news _details.php?fn=jul3013-text&yr=2013.

Johnson, Richard W., and Corina Mommaerts, for the Urban Institute. *Will Healthcare Costs Bankrupt Aging Boomers?* Washington, DC: The Urban Institute, 2010. Accessed October 23, 2014. http://www.urban.org /uploadedpdf/412026_health_care_costs.pdf.

Johnson, Richard W., and Janice S. Park. "Who Purchases Long-Term Care Insurance?" *Urban Institute Older Americans' Economic Security* 29 (March 2011). Accessed October 16, 2014. http://www.urban.org /UploadedPDF/412324-Long-Term-Care-Insurance.pdf.

Jones, Abigail. "Some Retirees Opting for Campus Life." *New York Times*, December 3, 2010. Accessed October 20, 2014. http://newoldage.blogs .nytimes.com/2010/12/03/some-retirees-opting-for-campus-life/?_php =true&_type=blogs&_r=0.

Judson, Timothy J., Allan S. Detsky, and Matthew J. Press. "Encouraging Patients to Ask Questions: How to Overcome 'White-Coat Silence'." *Journal of the American Medical Association* 309, no. 22 (2013): 2325–2326.

Jung, Younbo, Koay Jing Li, Ng Sihui Janissa, Wong Li Chieh Gladys, and Kwan Min Lee. "Games for a Better Life: Effects of Playing Wii Games on the Well-Being of Seniors in a Long-Term Care Facility." *Proceedings of the Sixth Australasian Conference on Interactive Entertainment* Article No. 5 (2009).

Kaiser Family Foundation. "Average Number of Deficiencies per Certified Nursing Facility." Accessed October 21, 2014. http://kff.org/other /state-indicator/avg-of-nursing-facility-deficiencies/.

Kaiser Family Foundation. "Distribution of Certified Nursing Facility Residents by Primary Payer Source, 2010." Accessed October 21, 2014. http:// www.statehealthfacts.org/comparebar.jsp?ind=410&cat=8.

Kaiser Family Foundation. "Percent of Certified Nursing Facilities with Top Ten Deficiencies." Accessed October 21, 2014. http://kff.org/other /state-indicator/top-ten-nursing-facility-deficiencies/.

Kaiser Family Foundation. "Total Number of Residents in Certified Nursing Facilities, 2010." Accessed October 21, 2014. http://www.statehealthfacts .org/comparemaptable.jsp?cat=8&ind=408.

Kaleem, Jaweed. "Death over Dinner, the Conversation Project Aim to Spark Discussions about the End of Life." *Huffington Post*, December 23, 2013. Accessed October 21, 2014. http://www.huffingtonpost.com/2013/12/23 /death-over-dinner-conversation-project_n_4495250.html.

Kaplan, Eve. "New Financial Burden for Boomers: Forced to Pay Parents' Long-Term-Care Costs." *Forbes*, August 13, 2012. Accessed October 16, 2014. http://www.forbes.com/sites/feeonlyplanner/2012/08/13

/new-financial-burden-for-boomers-forced-to-pay-parents-long-term -care-bill/.

Kaplan, Nicole, and Monika White, for the Center for Healthy Aging. *Getting Around: Alternatives for Seniors Who No Longer Drive*. Washington, DC: AAA Foundation for Traffic Safety, 2007. Accessed October 21, 2014. https://www.aaafoundation.org/sites/default/files/GettingAroundReport .pdf.

Karla, Nidhi, James Anderson, and Martin Wachs. *Liability and Regulation of Autonomous Vehicle Technologies: California PATH Research Report UCB-ITS-PRR-2009-28*. Arlington, VA: RAND, 2009. Accessed October 21, 2014. http://www.dot.ca.gov/newtech/researchreports/reports/2009 /prr-2009-28_liability_reg_&_auto_vehicle_final_report_2009.pdf.

Kassner, Enid. "Private Long-Term Care Insurance: The Medicaid Interaction." *AARP Issue Brief* 68 (2004). Accessed October 16, 2014. http://assets .aarp.org/rgcenter/health/ib68_ltc.pdf.

Kelley, Amy S., Susan L. Ettner, R. Sean Morrison, Qingling Du, Neil S. Wenger, and Catherine A. Sarkisian. "Determinants of Medical Expenditures in the Last 6 Months of Life." *Annals of Internal Medicine* 154, no. 4 (2011): 235–242.

Kelley, Amy S., Kathleen McGarry, Sean Fahle, Samuel M. Marshall, Qingling Du, and Jonathan S. Skinner. "Out-of-Pocket Spending in the Last Five Years of Life." *Journal of General Internal Medicine* 28, no. 2 (2013): 304–309.

Kelly, Anne, Jessamyn Conell-Price, Kenneth Covinsky, Irena Stijacic Cenzer, Anna Chang, W. John Boscardin, and Alexander K. Smith. "Length of Stay for Older Adults Residing in Nursing Homes at the End of Life." *Journal of American Geriatrics Society* 58, no. 9 (2010): 1701–1706.

Kim, Seongsu, and Daniel C. Feldman. "Working in Retirement: The Antecedents of Bridge Employment and Its Consequences for Quality of Life in Retirement." *Academy of Management Journal* 43, no. 6 (2000): 1195–1210.

King, Patricia A., Lawrence O. Gostin, and Judith C. Areen. *Law, Medicine and Ethics*. New York: Foundation Press, 2006.

Koerth-Baker, Maggie. "Death of a Caveman: What Swedish Babies and the Stone Age Can Teach Us about Life Expectancy and Income Inequality." *New York Times Magazine*, March 24, 2013, 14.

Kolata, Gina. "Dementia Rate Is Found to Drop Sharply, as Forecast." *New York Times*, June 16, 2013. Accessed October 16, 2014. http://www.nytimes .com/2013/07/17/health/study-finds-dip-in-dementia-rates.html?_r=0.

Konrad, Walecia. "Old, Infirm and at the Center of a Legal Struggle." *New York Times*, November 13, 2012. Accessed October 20, 2014. http://www .nytimes.com/2012/11/14/your-money/old-infirm-and-in-the-center-of-a -lawsuit.html?gwh=421D6CFD2852591EF9998620ABDDC488&gwt=pay.

KPMG. *Self-Driving Cars: The Next Revolution*. KPMG and Center for Automotive Research, 2012. Accessed October 21, 2014. https://www.kpmg .com/US/en/IssuesAndInsights/ArticlesPublications/Documents/self -driving-cars-next-revolution.pdf.

Kulikov, Elena. "The Social and Policy Predictors of Driving Mobility among Older Adults." *Journal of Aging & Social Policy* 23, no. 1 (2011): 1–18.

Kyle, Peter. "Confronting the Elder Care Crisis: The Private Long-Term Care Insurance Market and the Utility of Hybrid Products," *Marquette Elder's Advisor*, 15 (2013): 101–133.

Langford, Jim, Michael Fitzharris, Stuart Newstead, and Sjaanie Koppel. "Some Consequences of Different Older Driver Licensing Procedures in Australia." *Accident Analysis & Prevention* 36, no. 6 (2004): 993–1001.

Larson, Eric B., Kristine Yaffe, and Kenneth M. Langa. "New Insights into the Dementia Epidemic." *New England Journal of Medicine* 369 (2013): 2275–2277.

LearnVest. Accessed October 16, 2014. https://www.learnvest.com/.

Lee, Emily Oshima, and Ezekiel J. Emanuel. "Shared Decision Making to Improve Care and Reduce Costs." *New England Journal of Medicine* 368 (2013): 6–8.

LegalZoom. Accessed October 20, 2014. http://www.legalzoom.com.

Levi, Benjamin H., and Michael J. Green. "Too Soon to Give Up: Re-Examining the Value of Advance Directives." *American Journal of Bioethics* 10, no. 4 (2010): 3–22.

LIMRA. "Most Middle-Income Workers Saving Less than Five Percent of Their Income for Retirement." October 31, 2012. Accessed October 16, 2014. http://www.limra.com/Posts/PR/News_Releases/Most_Middle -Income_Workers_Saving_Less_Than_Five_Percent_of_Their_Income _for_Retirement.aspx.

Lopez, Ricardo. "Putting Off Retirement Cuts Chances of Dementia, Study Says." *Los Angeles Times*, July 15, 2013. Accessed October 21, 2014. http://www.latimes.com/business/money/la-fi-mo-retirement-dementia -study-20130715,0,5992576.story.

Ludwig, Wolfram, Klaus-Hendrik Wolf, Christopher Duwenkamp, Nathalie Gusew, Nils Hellrung, Michael Marschollek, Markus Wagner, and Reinhold Haux. "Health-Enabling Technologies for the Elderly—An Overview of Services Based on a Literature Review." *Computer Methods and Programs in Biomedicine* 106, no. 2 (2012): 70–78.

Lunney, June R., Joanne Lynn, Daniel J. Foley, Steven Lipson, and Jack M. Guralnik. "Patterns of Functional Decline at the End of Life." *Journal of the American Medical Association* 289, no. 18 (May 2003): 2387–2392.

Lunney, June R., Joanne Lynn, and Christopher Hogan. "Profiles of Older Medicare Decedents." *Journal of the American Geriatrics Society* 50, no. 6 (2002): 1108–1112.

Markoff, John. "Collision in the Making Between Self-Driving Cars and How the World Works." *New York Times*, January 23, 2011. Accessed October 21, 2014. http://www.nytimes.com/2012/01/24/technology/googles-autonomous-vehicles-draw-skepticism-at-legal-symposium.html?_r=0.

Markoff, John, and Somini Sengupta. "Drivers with Hands Full Get a Backup: The Car." *New York Times*, January 12, 2013. Accessed October 21, 2014. http://www.nytimes.com/2013/01/12/science/drivers-with-hands-full-get-a-backup-the-car.html?pagewanted=all.

Maryland State Advisory Council on Quality Care at the End of Life. *Study on a Statewide Advance Directive Registry* (2005). Accessed October 20, 2014. http://www.oag.state.md.us/Healthpol/ADregistry.pdf.

Mather LifeWays Institute on Aging, Ziegler, and Brecht Associates, Inc. *Final Report of National Survey of Family Members of Residents Living in Continuing Care Retirement Communities* (2011). Accessed October 20, 2014. http://www.nxtbook.com/nxtbooks/mather/finalreport2011/#/18.

Matthews, Fiona E., Antony Arthur, Linda E. Barnes, John Bond, Carol Jagger, Louise Robinson, and Carol Brayne, on behalf of the Medical Research Council Cognitive Function and Ageing Collaboration. "A Two-Decade Comparison of Prevalence of Dementia in Individuals Aged 65 Years and Older from Three Geographical Areas of England: Results of the Cognitive Function and Ageing Study I and II." *Lancet* 382, no. 9902 (2013): 1405–1412. Accessed October 16, 2014. http://download.thelancet.com/flatcontentassets/pdfs/S0140673613615706.pdf.

Mayo Clinic Staff. "Mediterranean Diet: A Heart-Healthy Eating Plan." Mayo Clinic. Accessed October 16, 2014. http://www.mayoclinic.com/health/mediterranean-diet/CL00011.

Meals on Wheels Association of America. "About MOWAA." Accessed October 20, 2014. http://www.mowaa.org/aboutus.

Medicaid.gov. "Find a Home Health Agency." Accessed November 2, 2014. http://www.medicare.gov/homehealthcompare/search.html.

Medicaid.gov. "Glossary-B." Accessed October 21, 2014. http://www.medicare.gov/glossary/b.html.

Medicaid.gov. "Spousal Impoverishment." Accessed November 2, 2014. http://www.medicaid.gov/Medicaid-CHIP-Program-Information/By-Topics/Eligibility/Spousal-Impoverishment-Page.html.

Medicare.gov. "Nursing Home Compare." Accessed October 21, 2014. http://www.medicare.gov/nursinghomecompare/search.html.

Menack, Julie. "Technologies That Support Aging in Place." In *Handbook of Geriatric Care Management*, edited by Cathy Jo Cress. Burlington, MA: Jones & Bartlett Learning, 2011.

Menzel, Paul T., and M. Colette Chandler-Cramer. "Advance Directives, Dementia, and Withholding Food and Water by Mouth." *Hastings Center Report* 44, no. 3 (2014): 23–37.

Mercer, Marsha. "How to Beat the Doctor Shortage." *AARP Bulletin*, March 2013. Accessed October 21, 2014. http://www.aarp.org/health/medicare-insurance/info-03-2013/how-to-beat-doctor-shortage.html.

MetLife Mature Market Institute, National Adult Day Service Association, and Ohio State University College of Social Work. *The MetLife National Study of Adult Day Services: Providing Support to Individuals and Their Family Caregiver.* New York: MetLife Mature Market Institute, 2010. Accessed October 21, 2014. https://www.metlife.com/assets/cao/mmi/publications/studies/2010/mmi-adult-day-services.pdf.

Michon, Kathleen. "Daily Money Management Programs for Seniors." *Nolo.* Accessed October 16, 2014. http://www.nolo.com/legal-encyclopedia/daily-money-management-programs-seniors-32269.html.

Miguel, Kristen De San, and Gill Lewin. "Personal Emergency Alarms: What Impact Do They Have on Older People's Lives?" *Australasian Journal on Ageing* 27, no. 2 (2008): 103–105.

Miles, C. J. "Concierge Medicine: An Alternative to Insurance." *Association of Mature American Citizens Health & Wealth*, June 26, 2014. Accessed November 6, 2014. http://amac.us/concierge-medicine-alternative-insurance/.

Moneychimp. "Simple Retirement Calculator." Accessed October 16, 2014. http://www.moneychimp.com/calculator/retirement_calculator.htm.

Monte, Lindsay M., and Renee R. Ellis. "Fertility of Women in the United States: 2012." *United States Census Population Characteristics* P20-575, July 2014. Accessed November 10, 2014. http://www.census.gov/content/dam/Census/library/publications/2014/demo/p20-575.pdf.

Morgan, Rebecca C. "The Future of Elder Law Practice." *William Mitchell Law Review* 37, no. 1 (2010): 1–49.

Morita, Ayako, Takehito Takano, Keiko Nakamura, Masashi Kizuki, and Kaoruko Seino. "Contribution of Interaction with Family, Friends and Neighbours, and Sense of Neighbourhood Attachment to Survival in Senior Citizens: 5-Year Follow-Up Study." *Social Science and Medicine* 70, no. 4 (2009): 543–549.

Muller, David. "Physician-Assisted Death Is Illegal in Most States, So My Patient Made Another Choice." *Health Affairs* 31, no. 10 (2012): 2343–2346.

Nasvadi, Glenyth E., and John Vavrik. "Crash Risk of Older Drivers after Attending a Mature Driver Education Program." *Accident Analysis & Prevention* 39, no. 6 (2007): 1073–1079.

National Academy of Elder Law Attorneys. "NAELA's History." Accessed November 25, 2014. http://www.naela.org/Public/About/Fact_Sheet/NAELA_s_History/Public/About_NAELA/History.aspx?hkey=8b2aab86-18e9-48cb-af8d-6afadee9f0f4.

National Adult Day Services Association. "The National Voice for the Adult Day Service Community." Accessed October 21, 2014. http://www.nadsa.org/.

National Adult Day Services Association. "Site Visit Checklist." Accessed October 21, 2014. http://nadsa.org/consumers/site-visit-checklist/.

National Adult Day Services Association. "State/International Association Partners." Accessed October 21, 2014. http://www.azularc.com/Development/nadsa/membership/state-association-partners/.

National Association of Insurance Commissioners. *Buyer's Guide to Long-Term Care Insurance.* Kansas City, MO: National Association of Insurance Commissioners, 2013.

National Association of Professional Geriatric Care Managers. "Find a Care Manager." Accessed October 16, 2014. http://memberfinder.caremanager.org/.

National Association of Professional Geriatric Care Managers. "What You Need to Know." Accessed October 16, 2014. http://www.caremanager.org/why-care-management/what-you-should-know/.

National Association of Professional Organizers. "Our Profession." Accessed October 16, 2014. http://www.napo.net/our_profession/.

National Center for Medical-Legal Partnership. "The Model." Accessed October 21, 2014. http://www.medical-legalpartnership.org/model.

National Council on Aging. "Senior Centers: Fact Sheet." Accessed October 21, 2014. http://www.ncoa.org/press-room/fact-sheets/senior-centers-fact-sheet.html.

National Elder Law Foundation. "About NELF." Accessed December 2, 2014. http://www.nelf.org/about-nelf.

National Elder Law Foundation. "Find a CELA." Accessed November 9, 2014. http://www.nelf.org/find-a-cela.

National Health Policy Forum. *Older Americans Act of 1965: Programs and Funding.* Washington, DC: National Health Policy Forum, 2012. Accessed October 21, 2014. http://www.nhpf.org/library/the-basics/Basics_OlderAmericansAct_02-23-12.pdf.

National Highway Traffic Safety Administration. *Traffic Safety Facts 2012: A Compilation of Motor Vehicle Crash Data from the Fatality Analysis Reporting System and the General Estimates System,* DOT HS 812 032. Washington, DC: National Highway Traffic Safety Administration, 2014. Accessed November 26, 2014. http://www-nrd.nhtsa.dot.gov/Pubs/812032.pdf.

National Hospice and Palliative Care Organization. *NHPCO's Facts and Figures: Hospice Care in America, 2014 Edition.* Alexandria, VA: National Hospice and Palliative Care Organization, 2014. Accessed November 5, 2014. http://www.nhpco.org/sites/default/files/public/Statistics_Research/2014_Facts_Figures.pdf.

National Resource Center on Psychiatric Advance Directives. "Do All States Specifically Have PAD Statutes?" Accessed October 20, 2014. http://www.nrc-pad.org/faqs/do-all-states-specifically-have-pad-statutes.

National Reverse Mortgage Lenders Association. "Your Guide to Reverse Mortgages." 2014. Accessed October 16, 2014. http://www.reversemortgage.org/.

National Shared Housing Resource Center. Accessed October 20, 2014. http://nationalsharedhousing.org/.

Naturally Occurring Retirement Community. "NORC: Georgia's Neighborhood Approach to Healthy Aging." Accessed October 20, 2014. http://www.tocohillsnorc.org/.

Negri, Kathleen A. "Advance Care Planning: The Attorney's Role in Helping Clients Achieve a 'Good Death'." *Colorado Lawyer* (July 2012): 67–76.

Nerenberg, Lisa. *Daily Money Management Programs: A Protection against Elder Abuse*. Washington, DC: National Center on Elder Abuse, 2003. Accessed October 16, 2014. http://www.ncea.aoa.gov/Resources/Publication/docs/DailyMoneyManagement.pdf.

Neuberg, Gerald W. "The Cost of End-of-Life Care: A New Efficiency Measure Falls Short of AHA/ACC Standards." *Cardiovascular Quality and Outcomes* 2, no. 2 (2009): 127–133.

Newbridge on the Charles. "Frequently Asked Questions." Accessed October 20, 2014. http://www.hebrewseniorlife.org/newbridge-frequently-asked-questions.

Newton, Michael J. "Precedent Autonomy: Life-Sustaining Intervention and the Demented Patient." *Cambridge Quarterly of Healthcare Ethics* 8, no. 2 (1999): 189–199.

Nonprofit Vote. *America Goes to the Polls 2012: A Report of Voter Turnout in the 2012 Election*. Boston, MA: Nonprofit VOTE. Accessed October 21, 2014. http://www.nonprofitvote.org/voter-turnout.html.

O'Brien, Elizabeth. "Know Your Retirement Community's Exit Options." *MarketWatch*, June 19, 2013. Accessed November 24, 2014. http://www.marketwatch.com/story/retirement-communities-read-the-contract-2013-06-19.

O'Brien, Elizabeth. "Why Concierge Medicine Will Get Bigger: Practices Could Shield Patients from Health-Care Turmoil." *MarketWatch*, January 17, 2013. Accessed October 21, 2014. http://www.aarp.org/health/healthy-living/info-01-2013/boutique-doctors.html.

Office of the Minnesota Attorney General. "Nursing Homes and Assisted Living." Accessed October 21, 2014. http://www.ag.state.mn.us/consumer/ylr/nursinghomesassistedliving.asp.

Ohio Legal Services. "Wills and Probate: Financial Power of Attorney." Accessed October 20, 2014. http://www.ohiolegalservices.org/public/legal_problem/wills-and-probate/financial-power-of-attorney/qandact_view.

Ohio State Bar Association. "What You Should Know about the Declaration of Mental Health Treatment." Accessed October 20, 2014. https://www.ohiobar.org/ForPublic/Resources/LawYouCanUse/Pages/LawYouCanUse-298.aspx.

Olson, Elizabeth. "Concerns Rise about Continuing-Care Enclaves." *New York Times*, September 15, 2010. Accessed October 20, 2014. http://www.nytimes.com/2010/09/16/business/retirementspecial/16CARE.html?pagewanted=all&_r=0.

Ong, Anthony D., Jeremy D. Rothstein, and Bert N. Uchino. "Loneliness Accentuates Age Differences in Cardiovascular Responses to Social Evaluative Threat." *Psychology and Aging* 27, no. 1 (2012): 190–198.

Oregon Public Health Division. "Oregon's Death with Dignity Act—2013." Accessed November 12, 2014. http://public.health.oregon.gov/ProviderPartnerResources/EvaluationResearch/DeathwithDignityAct/Documents/year16.pdf.

Organisation for Economic Co-operation and Development. *The Future of Families to 2030.* OECD Publishing, 2012. Accessed October 16, 2014. http://www.leavenetwork.org/fileadmin/Leavenetwork/News/Future_Families_2030.pdf.

Ortman, Jennifer M., Victoria A. Velkoff, and Howard Hogan. "An Aging Nation: The Older Population in the United States: Population Estimates and Projections." *United States Census Bureau Report* P25-1140, May 2014. Accessed November 7, 2014. https://www.census.gov/content/dam/Census/library/publications/2014/demo/p25-1140.pdf.

Owsley, Cynthia, Gerald McGwin Jr., Janice M. Phillips, Sandre F. McNeal, and Beth T. Stalvey. "Impact of an Educational Program on the Safety of High-Risk, Visually Impaired, Older Drivers." *American Journal of Preventive Medicine* 26, no. 3 (2004): 222–229.

Parikh, Ravi B., Rebecca A. Kirch, Thomas J. Smith, and Jennifer S. Temel. "Early Specialty Palliative Care—Translating Data in Oncology into Practice." *New England Journal of Medicine* 369, no. 24 (2013): 2347–2351.

Parker, Kim, and Eileen Patten. "The Sandwich Generation: Rising Financial Burdens for Middle-Aged Americans." *Pew Research Center Social & Demographic Trends*, January 30, 2013. Accessed October 16, 2014. http://www.pewsocialtrends.org/2013/01/30/the-sandwich-generation/.

Pearson, Katherine C. "Filial Support Laws in the Modern Era: Domestic and International Comparison of Enforcement Practices for Laws Requiring Adult Children to Support Indigent Parents." *Elder Law Journal* 20 (2013): 269–304.

Pergolizzi, Joseph, Rainer H. Böger, Keith Budd, Albert Dahan, Serdar Erdine, Guy Hans, Hans-Georg Kress, Richard Langford, Rudolf Likar,

Robert B. Raffa, and Paola Sacerdote. "Opioids and the Management of Chronic Severe Pain in the Elderly: Consensus Statement of an International Expert Panel with Focus on the Six Clinically Most Often Used World Health Organization Step III Opioids (Buprenorphine, Fentanyl, Hydromorphone, Methadone, Morphine, Oxycodone)." *Pain Practice* 8, no. 4 (2008): 287–311.

Perissinotto, Carla M., Irena Stijacic Cenzer, and Kenneth E. Covinsky. "Loneliness in Older Persons: A Predictor of Functional Decline and Death." *Archives of Internal Medicine* 172, no. 44 (2012): 1078–1083.

Peterson, Lars E., Andrew Bazemore, Elizabeth J. Bragg, Imam Xierali, and Gregg A. Warshaw. "Rural-Urban Distribution of the U.S. Geriatrics Physician Workforce." *Journal of the American Geriatrics Society* 59, no. 4 (2011): 699–703.

Petterson, Stephen M., Winston R. Liaw, Robert L. Phillips Jr., David L. Rabin, David S. Meyers, and Andrew W. Bazemore. "Projecting US Primary Care Physician Workforce Needs: 2010–2025." *Annals of Family Medicine* 10, no. 6 (2012): 503–509.

Pew Research Center. *Angry Silents, Disengaged Millennials: The Generation Gap and the 2012 Election.* Washington, DC: Pew Research Center, 2011. Accessed October 21, 2014. http://www.people-press.org/files/legacy -pdf/11-3-11%20Generations%20Release.pdf.

Pew Research Center. "Attitudes about Aging: A Global Perspective." *Pew Research Global Attitudes Project*, January 30, 2014. Accessed October 16, 2014. http://www.pewglobal.org/2014/01/30/attitudes-about-aging-a -global-perspective/.

Pew Research Center. *Baby Boomers Retire.* Washington, DC: Pew Research Center, 2010. Accessed October 21, 2014. http://www.pewresearch.org /daily-number/baby-boomers-retire.

Pew Research Center. "Views on End-of-Life Medical Treatments." *Pew Research Religion & Public Life Project*, November 21, 2013. Accessed October 21, 2014. http://www.pewforum.org/2013/11/21/views-on-end-of -life-medical-treatments/.

Physician Orders for Life Sustaining Treatment Paradigm. "Programs in Your State." Accessed October 21, 2014. http://www.polst.org/programs -in-your-state/.

Pillemer, Karl, and Nina Glasgow. "Social Integration and Aging: Background and Trends." In *Social Integration in the Second Half of Life*, edited by Karl Pillemer, Phyllis Moen, Elaine Wethington, and Nina Glasgow, 19–47. Baltimore, MD: Johns Hopkins University Press, 2000.

Population Reference Bureau. "Social Support, Networks, and Happiness." *Today's Research on Aging* 17 (2009): 1–6.

Post, Stephen G. "Alzheimer Disease and the 'Then' Self." *Kennedy Institute of Ethics Journal* 5, no. 4 (1995): 307–321.

ProPublica. Accessed October 20, 2014. http://www.propublica.org/about/.

ProviderData. "Calaroga Terrace." Accessed October 20, 2014. http://www
.providerdata.com/portland-or/167258/calaroga-terrace.aspx.

Rauch, Jonathan. "How Not to Die." *Atlantic*, April 24, 2013. Accessed
October 21, 2014. http://www.theatlantic.com/magazine/archive/2013/05
/how-not-to-die/309277/.

Richardson, Derek K., Dana Zive, Mohamud Daya, and Craig D. Newgard.
"The Impact of Early Do Not Resuscitate (DNR) Orders on Patient Care
and Outcomes Following Resuscitation from Out of Hospital Cardiac
Arrest." *Resuscitation* 84, no. 4 (2013): 483–487.

Riley, Gerald F., and James D. Lubitz. "Long-Term Trends in Medicare Payments in the Last Year of Life." *Health Services Research* 45, no. 2 (2010):
565–576.

Rosenblatt, Carolyn. "The Hidden Truths about Reverse Mortgages."
Forbes, July 23, 2012. Accessed October 16, 2014. http://www.forbes
.com/sites/carolynrosenblatt/2012/07/23/hidden-truths-about-reverse
-mortgages/2.

Roth, J. D. "How Much Should You Save for Retirement?" *Time*, December
5, 2012. Accessed October 16, 2014. http://business.time.com/2012/12/05
/how-much-should-you-save-for-retirement/.

Rowe, John Wallis, and Robert Louis Kahn. *Successful Aging*. New York: Dell
Publishing, 1998.

Rubin, Gretchen. *The Happiness Project: Or, Why I Spent a Year Trying to Sing
in the Morning, Clean My Closets, Fight Right, Read Aristotle, and Generally Have More Fun*. New York: HarperCollins, 2009.

Rubin, Joel, Daren Briscoe, and Mitchell Landsberg. "Car Plows Through
Crowd in Santa Monica, Killing 9." *Los Angeles Times*, July 17, 2003.
Accessed October 21, 2014. http://articles.latimes.com/2003/jul/17/local
/me-smcrash17.

Russo, Richard. *Elsewhere*. New York: Knopf, 2012.

Sabatino, Charles P. "Damage Prevention and Control for Financial Incapacity." *Journal of the American Medical Association* 305, no. 7 (2011):
707–708.

Sacks, Debra, Dhiman Das, Raquel Romanick, Matt Caron, Carmen Morano,
and Marianne C. Fahs. "The Value of Daily Money Management: An
Analysis of Outcomes and Costs." *Journal of Evidence-Based Social Work*
9, no. 5 (2012): 498–511.

Sanders, Bernard, Subcommittee on Primary Health and Aging, U.S. Senate Committee on Health, Education, Labor & Pensions. *Primary Care
Access: 30 Million New Patients and 11 Months to Go: Who Will Provide
Their Primary Care?* U.S. Senate, 2013. Accessed October 21, 2014. http://
www.sanders.senate.gov/imo/media/doc/PrimaryCareAccessReport
.pdf.

Scharlach, Andrew, Carrie Graham, and Amanda Lehning. "The 'Village' Model: A Consumer-Driven Approach for Aging in Place." *The Gerontologist* 52, no. 3 (2011): 418–427.

Scott, Lisa M., and Candace Sharkey. "Putting the Pieces Together: Private-Duty Home Healthcare and Geriatric Care Management: One Home Health Agency's Model." *Home Healthcare Nurse* 25, no. 3 (2007): 167–172.

SeniorHomes.com. "55+ Communities." Accessed October 20, 2014. http://www.seniorhomes.com/p/55-communities/.

Shah, Neil. "More Young Adults Live with Parents." *Wall Street Journal*, August 27, 2013. Accessed October 16, 2014. http://online.wsj.com/news/articles/SB10001424127887324906304579039313087064716.

Shapiro, Susan P. "Advance Directives: The Elusive Goal of Having the Last Word." *Journal of the National Academy of Elder Law Attorneys* 8, no. 2 (2012): 204–232.

Shugarman, Lisa R., Sandra L. Decker, and Anita Bercovitz. "Demographic and Social Characteristics and Spending at the End of Life." *Journal of Pain and Symptom Management* 38, no. 1 (2009): 15–26.

Shulevitz, Judith. "Why Do Grandmothers Exist?" *The New Republic*, January 29, 2013. Accessed October 20, 2014. http://www.newrepublic.com/article/112199/genetics-grandmothers-why-they-exist.

Silveira, Maria J., Scott Y. H. Kim, and Kenneth M. Langa. "Advance Directives and Outcomes of Surrogate Decision Making before Death." *New England Journal of Medicine* 362 (2010): 1211–1218.

Simon, Nissa. "Is a 'Boutique' Doctor for You? Here's What You Need to Know Before Signing Up with a 'Concierge' Practice." *AARP Health*, January 7, 2013. Accessed October 21, 2014. http://www.aarp.org/health/healthy-living/info-01-2013/boutique-doctors.html.

Sinha, Sahab P., P. Nayyar, and Surat P. Sinha. "Social Support and Self-Control as Variables in Attitude toward Life and Perceived Control among Older People in India." *Journal of Social Psychology* 142, no. 4 (2002): 527–540.

Sloane, Kelly Lauren. "If Only Grown-Ups Would Pay Attention." *Journal of the American Medical Association* 309, no. 8 (2013): 779–780.

Sommerfeld, Lorraine. "Drive, She Said: New Test Coming Soon for Elderly Ontario Drivers." *The Globe and Mail*, January 31, 2014. Accessed October 21, 2014. http://www.theglobeandmail.com/globe-drive/news/new-test-coming-soon-for-elderly-ontario-drivers/article16638607/.

Span, Paula. "A Better Way to Find Home Care Aides." *New York Times*, May 4, 2011. Accessed October 21, 2014. http://newoldage.blogs.nytimes.com/2011/05/04/a-better-way-to-find-home-care-aides/.

Span, Paula. "Help by the Hour, or Less." *New York Times*, November 23, 2012. Accessed November 1, 2014. http://newoldage.blogs.nytimes.com/2012/11/23/1123-help-by-the-hour/?_r=0.

Span, Paula. "Now, Tables for (Almost) Everyone." *New York Times*, March 6, 2012. Accessed October 20, 2014. http://newoldage.blogs.nytimes.com/2012/03/06/now-tables-for-almost-everyone/.

Span, Paula. "Two Kinds of Hospital Patients: Admitted, and Not." *New York Times*, October 29, 2013. Accessed October 21, 2014. http://newoldage.blogs.nytimes.com/2013/10/29/two-kinds-of-hospital-patients-admitted-and-not/.

Span, Paula. *When the Time Comes: Families with Aging Parents Share Their Struggles and Solutions.* New York: Springboard Press, 2009.

Starfield, Barbara, Hsien-Yen Chang, Klaus W. Lemke, and Jonathan P. Weine. "Ambulatory Specialist Use by Nonhospitalized Patients in US Health Plans: Correlates and Consequences." *Journal of Ambulatory Care Management* 32, no. 3 (2009): 216–225.

Starfield, Barbara, Klaus W. Lemke, Robert Herbert, Wendy D. Pavlovich, and Gerard Anderson. "Comorbidity and the Use of Primary Care and Specialist Care in the Elderly." *Annals of Family Medicine* 3, no. 3 (2005): 215–222.

State of Connecticut Office of the Treasurer. "Office of Connecticut State Treasurer Denise L. Nappier and Financial Planning Associations of Connecticut Announce the FPA CT Pro Bono Network." *Office of CT State Treasurer News*, November 10, 2008. Accessed October 16, 2014. http://www.ott.ct.gov/pressreleases/press2008/PR11102008.pdf.

Suryadevara, N. K., S. C. Mukhopadhyay, R. K. Rayudu, and Y. M. Huang. "Sensor Data Fusion to Determine Wellness of an Elderly in Intelligent Home Monitoring Environment." *Instrumentation and Measurement Technology Conference (I2MTC), 2012 IEEE International* (2012): 947–952.

Swan, Beth Ann. "A Nurse Learns Firsthand That You May Fend for Yourself After a Hospital Stay." *Health Affairs* 31, no. 11 (2012): 2579–2582.

Takacs, Timothy L. "The Life Care Plan: Integrating a Healthcare-Focused Approach to Meeting the Needs of Your Clients and Families into Your Elder Law Practice." *NAELA Quarterly* 16 (2003): 2–8.

Tchirkow, Paula P. "Advocates for the Elderly and 'Eyes and Ears' for Elder Law Attorneys." *Pennsylvania Lawyer* 24 (2002): 34–37.

Tefft, Brian. "Risks Older Drivers Pose to Themselves and to Other Road Users." *Journal of Safety Research* 39, no. 6 (2008): 577–582.

Temel, Jennifer S., Joseph A. Greer, Alona Muzikansky, Emily R. Gallagher, Sonal Admane, Vicki A. Jackson, Constance M. Dahlin, Craig D. Blinderman, Juliet Jacobsen, William F. Pirl, J. Andrew Billings, and Thomas J. Lynch. "Early Palliative Care for Patients with Metastatic Non–Small-Cell Lung Cancer." *New England Journal of Medicine* 363, no. 8 (2010): 733–742.

Tergesen, Anne. "A Little Help with the Bills." *Wall Street Journal*, July 27, 2012. Accessed October 16, 2014. http://online.wsj.com/articles/SB100008 72396390444840104577550910299244458.

Terman, Stanley A. "It Isn't Easy Being Pink: Potential Problems with POLST Paradigm Forms." *Hamline Law Review* 36, no. 2 (2013): 177–211.

Thaler, Richard H., and Cass R. Sunstein. *Nudge: Improving Decisions about Health, Wealth, and Happiness.* New York: Penguin, 2009.

Thomas, Irene M. "Childless by Choice: Why Some Latinas Are Saying No to Motherhood." *Hispanic* 8, no. 4 (May 1995): 50.

Tomaka, Joe, Sharon Thompson, and Rebecca Palacios. "The Relation of Social Isolation, Loneliness, and Social Support to Disease Outcomes among the Elderly." *Journal of Aging and Health* 18, no. 3 (2006): 359–384.

Tomita, Machiko R., Linda S. Russ, Ramalingam Sridhar, and Bruce J. Naughton. *Smart Home with Healthcare Technologies for Community-Dwelling Older Adults.* In Tech, 2010. Accessed October 21, 2014. http://cdn .intechopen.com/pdfs/9628/InTech-Smart_home_with_healthcare _technologies_for_community_dwelling_older_adults.pdf.

Tommasulo, Peter. *Advance Directive Registries: A Policy Opportunity.* Center for Healthcare Research and Transformation, 2011. Accessed October 20, 2014. http://www.chrt.org/public-policy/policy-papers/advance -directive-registries-a-policy-opportunity/.

Triplett, Patrick, Betty S. Black, Hilary Phillips, Sarah Richardson Fahrendorf, Jack Schwartz, Andrew F. Angelino, Danielle Anderson, and Peter V. Rabins. "Content of Advance Directives for Individuals with Advanced Dementia." *Journal of Aging and Health* 20, no. 5 (2008): 583–596.

Tyrrell, Kelly April. "Delays, Controversy Muddle CMS' Two-Midnight Rule for Hospital Patient Admissions." *The Hospitalist*, April 2014. Accessed November 2, 2014. http://www.the-hospitalist.org/details/article/6020631 /Delays_Controversy_Muddle_CMS_Two-Midnight_Rule_for_Hospital _Patient_Admissions.html.

Uniform Law Commission. "Power of Attorney." Accessed October 20, 2014. http://www.uniformlaws.org/Act.aspx?title=Power%20of%20Attorney.

University of Minnesota Long-Term Care Resource Center. "NH Regulations Plus: State Regulation by State." Last modified March 19, 2012. Accessed October 20, 2014. http://www.hpm.umn.edu/nhregsplus/NHRegs_by _State/By%20State%20Main.html.

U.S. Census Bureau. "10 Percent of Grandparents Live with a Grandchild, Census Bureau Reports." *United States Census Bureau News Release.* Number: CB 14-194, October 22, 2014. Accessed October 22, 2014. http:// www.census.gov/newsroom/press-releases/2014/cb14-194.html.

U.S. Congressional Budget Office Cost Estimate. *S. 1562 Older Americans Act Reauthorization Act of 2013: As Reported by the Senate Committee on Health, Education, Labor, and Pensions on January 6.* Washington, DC:

Congressional Budget Office Cost Estimate, 2014. Accessed October 21, 2014. http://www.cbo.gov/sites/default/files/s1562.pdf.

U.S. Department of Health and Human Services. "Donate the Gift of Life." Accessed October 20, 2014. http://www.organdonor.gov/index.html.

U.S. Department of Health and Human Services. *Health, United States, 2013 with Special Feature on Prescription Drugs.* Hyattsville, MD: 2014. Accessed November 20, 2014. http://www.cdc.gov/nchs/data/hus/hus13.pdf.

U.S. Department of Health and Human Services. "Secretary Sebelius' Letter to Congress about CLASS." October 14, 2011. Accessed October 16, 2014. http://www.ltcconsultants.com/articles/2011/class-dismissed/Sebelius -CLASS-Letter.pdf.

U.S. Department of Health and Human Services, Administration on Aging & Administration for Community Living. "A Profile of Older Americans: 2013." Accessed November 10, 2014. http://www.aoa.acl.gov/Aging _Statistics/Profile/2013/docs/2013_Profile.pdf.

U.S. Department of Health and Human Services, National Center on Elder Abuse, Administration on Aging. "Statistics/Data." Accessed October 21, 2014. http://www.ncea.aoa.gov/Library/Data/index.aspx#oblem.

U.S. Department of Health and Human Services, Office of the Assistant Secretary for Planning and Evaluation (ASPE). *Advance Directives and Advance Care Planning: Report to Congress.* Washington, DC: ASPE, August 2008. Accessed October 20, 2014. http://aspe.hhs.gov/daltcp/reports/2008 /ADCongRpt.pdf.

U.S. Department of Health and Human Services, Office of Inspector General. *Adverse Events in Skilled Nursing Facilities: National Incidence among Medicare Beneficiaries.* Washington, DC: Office of Inspector General, 2014. Accessed October 21, 2014. http://oig.hhs.gov/oei/reports /oei-06-11-00370.pdf.

U.S. Department of Labor. "Retirement Plans, Benefits & Savings, Types of Plans." Accessed October 17, 2014. http://www.dol.gov/dol/topic/retire- ment/typesofplans.htm.

U.S. Department of Labor, Bureau of Labor Statistics. "Occupational Employment and Wages, May 2012, Home Health Aides." Accessed October 21, 2014. http://www.bls.gov/oes/current/oes311011.htm.

U.S. Government Accountability Office. *Older Americans: Continuing Care Retirement Communities Can Provide Benefits, but Not without Some Risk* (2010). Accessed October 20, 2014. http://www.gao.gov/new.items/d10611 .pdf.

USLegal. Accessed October 20, 2014. http://www.uslegalforms.com /wills/?auslf=buildawill.

U.S. Living Will Registry. "Frequently Asked Questions (FAQ) about the U.S. Living Will Registry." Accessed October 20, 2014. http://www .uslivingwillregistry.com/faq.shtm.

U.S. Securities and Exchange Commission. "Transfer on Death (TOD) Registration." Accessed October 20, 2014. http://www.sec.gov/answers /todreg.htm.

U.S. Senate. *Statement of Thomas E. Hamilton, Director, Survey and Certification Group, Center for Medicaid and State Operations, Centers for Medicare & Medicaid Services on Making the Case for Long-Term Care Services and Supports Before the Senate Special Committee on Aging.* U.S. Senate, March 4, 2009. Accessed October 21, 2014. http://www.aging.senate.gov/ imo/media/doc/hr205th.pdf.

U.S. Senate Special Committee on Aging. *Continuing Care Retirement Communities: Risks to Seniors: Summary of Committee Investigation* (2010). Accessed October 20, 2014. http://riverwoodsrc.org/sites/default/files /PDFs/Senate_Report.pdf.

U.S. Social Security Administration. "Fact Sheet: Social Security." Accessed October 16, 2014. http://www.ssa.gov/pressoffice/factsheets/basicfact-alt .pdf.

U.S. Social Security Administration. "Retirement Calculator: Full Retirement Age." Accessed October 16, 2014. http://www.ssa.gov/retire2/retirechart .htm.

U.S. Social Security Administration. "Social Security Retirement Benefits." *Social Security Administration Publication* No. 05-10035 (April 2013). Accessed October 21, 2014. http://www.ssa.gov/pubs/EN-05-10035.pdf.

Vaillant, George E. *Aging Well: Surprising Guideposts to a Happier Life from the Landmark Harvard Study of Adult Development.* Boston: Little Brown and Company, 2002.

Vance, Ashlee. "Why Do Hearing Aids Cost More Than Laptops?" *Bloomberg Busineessweek Technology,* June 6, 2013. Accessed October 16, 2014. http://www.businessweek.com/articles/2013-06-06/why-do-hearing -aids-cost-more-than-laptops.

Vanderbilt, Tom. "Let the Robot Drive: The Autonomous Car of the Future Is Here." *Wired Magazine,* January 20, 2012. Accessed October 21, 2014. http://www.wired.com/magazine/2012/01/ff_autonomouscars.

Vogel, T., P.-H. Brechat, P.-M. Lepretre, G. Kaltenbach, M. Berthel, and J. Lonsdorfer. "Health Benefits of Physical Activity in Older Patients: A Review." *International Journal of Clinical Practice* 63, no. 2 (2009): 303–320.

Wall Street Journal. "How to Choose a Financial Planner." December 17, 2008. Accessed October 16, 2014. http://guides.wsj.com/personal -finance/managing-your-money/how-to-choose-a-financial-planner/tab /print/.

Wall Street Journal. "Should You Purchase Long-Term-Care Insurance?" May 14, 2012. Accessed October 16, 2014. http://online.wsj.com/article/SB10001 424052702303425504577352031401783756.html.

Wang, Harry. "Tech Advances Will Give Aging Baby Boomers More Independence." *E-Commerce Times*, October 1, 2014. Accessed December 2, 2014. http://www.ecommercetimes.com/story/81128.html.

Warshaw, Gregg A., Elizabeth J. Bragg, and Ruth W. Shaull. *Geriatric Medicine Training and Practice in the United States at the Beginning of the 21st Century.* The Association of Directors of Geriatric Academic Programs, July 2002. Accessed October 20, 2014. http://www.americangeriatrics.org /files/documents/gwps/ADGAP%20Full%20Report.pdf.

Washington State Department of Health. "Washington State Department of Health 2013 Death with Dignity Act Report." Accessed November 12, 2014. http://www.doh.wa.gov/portals/1/Documents/Pubs/422-109 -DeathWithDignityAct2013.pdf.

Washington State Department of Social and Health Services. "Long-term Care Residential Options." Accessed October 21, 2014. http://www.altsa .dshs.wa.gov/pubinfo/housing/other/.

Weber, Tracy, Charles Ornstein, and Jennifer LaFleur. "Dangers Found in Lack of Safety Oversight for Medicare Drug Benefit." *Washington Post*, May 11, 2013. Accessed October 20, 2014. http://www.washingtonpost .com/national/health-science/dangers-found-in-lack-of-safety-oversight -for-medicare-drug-benefit/2013/05/11/067a10ae-b8ec-11e2-aa9e-a02b765 ff0ea_story.html.

Weisman, Steve. *A Guide to Elder Planning: Everything You Need to Know to Protect Your Loved Ones and Yourself.* Upper Saddle River, NJ: FT Press, 2013.

Weisman, Steve. *A Guide to Elder Planning: Everything You Need to Know to Protect Yourself Legally and Financially.* Upper Saddle River, NJ: Prentice Hall, 2004.

Wen, Leana, and Joshua Kosowsky. *When Doctors Don't Listen: How to Avoid Misdiagnoses and Unnecessary Tests.* New York: St. Martin's Press, 2012.

Wennberg, J. E., Elliott S. Fisher, David C. Goodman, and Jonathan S. Skinner. *Tracking the Course of Patients with Severe Chronic Illness: The Dartmouth Atlas of Health Care 2008*, edited by Kristen K. Bronner. Lebanon, NH: Dartmouth Institute for Health Policy & Clinical Practice, 2008. Accessed October 21, 2014. http://www.dartmouthatlas.org/downloads /atlases/2008_Chronic_Care_Atlas.pdf.

"When Five-Star Care Is Substandard: Medicare's Flawed Ratings for Nursing Homes." *New York Times*, August 25, 2014. Accessed November 2, 2014. http://www.nytimes.com/2014/08/26/opinion/medicares-flawed-ratings -for-nursing-homes.html?_r=0.

Whoriskey, Peter, and Dan Keating. "Dying and Profits: The Evolution of Hospice," *The Washington Post*, December 26, 2014, accessed February 7, 2015, http://www.washingtonpost.com/business/economy/2014/12/26 /a7d90438-692f-11e4-b053-65cea7903f2e_story.html.

Wideman, Marilyn. "Geriatric Care Management: Role, Need, and Benefits." *Home Healthcare Nurse* 30, no. 9 (2012): 553–559.

Widera, Eric, Veronika Steenpass, Daniel Marson, and Rebecca Sudore. "Finances in the Older Patient with Cognitive Impairment: 'He Didn't Want Me to Take Over'." *Journal of the American Medical Association* 305, no. 7 (2011): 698–706.

Winter, Michael. "100-Year-Old Driver Injures 9 Kids, 2 Adults Near School." *USA Today*, August 29, 2012. Accessed October 21, 2014. http://content.usatoday.com/communities/ondeadline/post/2012/08/driver-101-hits-parents-kids-outside-la-school-8-hurt/1.

Wolff, Michael. "A Life Worth Ending." *New York Magazine*, May 20, 2012. Accessed October 21, 2014. http://nymag.com/news/features/parent-health-care-2012-5/.

Women's Institute for Financial Education. "The People and Mission Behind Wife.org." Accessed October 16, 2014. http://www.wife.org.

Wu, Ya-Huei, Christine Fassert, and Anne-Sophie Rigaud. "Designing Robots for the Elderly: Appearance Issue and Beyond." *Archives of Gerontology and Geriatrics* 54, no. 1 (2012): 121–126.

Xu, Jiaquan, Kenneth D. Kochanek, Sherry L. Murphy, and Elizabeth Arias. "Mortality in the United States, 2012." *NCHS Data Brief* No. 168 (October 2014). Accessed November 10, 2014. http://www.cdc.gov/nchs/data/databriefs/db168.pdf.

Yarnall, Kimberly S. H., Truls Østbye, Katrina M. Krause, Kathryn I. Pollak, Margaret Gradison, and J. Lloyd Michener. "Family Physicians as Team Leaders: 'Time' to Share the Care." *Preventing Chronic Disease: Public Health Research, Practice, and Policy* 6, no. 2 (2009): A59. Accessed October 21, 2014. http://www.cdc.gov/pcd/issues/2009/apr/08_0023.htm.

Yuen, Jacqueline K., M. Carrington Reid, and Michael D. Fetters. "Hospital Do-Not-Resuscitate Orders: Why They Have Failed and How to Fix Them." *Journal of General Internal Medicine* 26, no. 7 (2011): 791–797.

Zamora, Enrique, Deborah Nodar, and Krista Ogletree. "Long-Term Care Insurance: A Life Raft for Baby Boomers," *Saint Thomas Law Review*, 26 (2013): 79–102.

Zarem, Jane E., ed. *Today's Continuing Care Retirement Community (CCRC)*. CCRC Task Force, July 2010. Accessed October 20, 2014. https://www.seniorshousing.org/filephotos/research/CCRC_whitepaper.pdf.

Zhong, Wenjun, Hilal Maradit-Kremers, Jennifer L. St. Sauver, Barbara P. Yawn, Jon O. Ebbert, Véronique L. Roger, Debra J. Jacobson, Michaela E. McGree, Scott M. Brue, and Walter A. Rocca. "Age and Sex Patterns of Drug Prescribing in a Defined American Population." *Mayo Clinic Proceedings* 88, no. 7 (2013): 697–707.

Zimmerman, Sheryl, Philip D. Sloane, J. Kevin Eckert, Ann L. Gruber-Baldini, Leslie A. Morgan, J. Richard Hebel, Jay Magaziner, Sally C. Stearns, and Cory K. Chen. "How Good Is Assisted Living? Findings and Implications from an Outcomes Study." *Journal of Gerontology Series B Psychological Sciences & Social Science* 60, no. 4 (2005): S195–S204.

Index

About the Author

Sharona Hoffman, J.D., LL.M., is the Edgar A. Hahn professor of law, professor of bioethics, and codirector of the Law School's Law-Medicine Center at Case Western Reserve University in Cleveland, Ohio. She received her B.A. magna cum laude from Wellesley College, her J.D. cum laude from Harvard Law School, and an LL.M. in health law from the University of Houston. She has twice spent a sabbatical semester as a visiting scholar at the Centers for Disease Control and Prevention (2007 and 2014) and was a Robert Wood Johnson Foundation fellow in public health law in 2013.

She has published over 60 articles and book chapters on a broad range of health law and discrimination issues. She has won several awards for teaching and scholarship. She has also lectured throughout the United States and internationally and has been widely featured in the media.